Operation Ebola

OPERATION HEALTH

A SERIES OF BOOKS EXPLORING SURGERY AND GLOBAL HEALTH

Operation Ebola

Surgical Care during the
West African Outbreak

EDITED BY

Sherry M. Wren, MD, FACS, FCS(ECSA)
STANFORD UNIVERSITY

AND

Adam L. Kushner, MD, MPH, FACS
JOHNS HOPKINS BLOOMBERG SCHOOL
OF PUBLIC HEALTH

FOREWORD BY

David B. Hoyt, MD, FACS
EXECUTIVE DIRECTOR
AMERICAN COLLEGE OF SURGEONS

JOHNS HOPKINS UNIVERSITY PRESS   BALTIMORE

© 2017 Johns Hopkins University Press
All rights reserved. Published 2017
Printed in the United States of America on acid-free paper
9 8 7 6 5 4 3 2 1

Johns Hopkins University Press
2715 North Charles Street
Baltimore, Maryland 21218-4363
www.press.jhu.edu

Library of Congress Cataloging-in-Publication Data

Names: Wren, Sherry M., 1960– editor. | Kushner, Adam L., 1965– editor.
Title: Operation Ebola : surgical care during the West African outbreak /
    [edited by] Sherry M. Wren and Adam L. Kushner.
Other titles: Operation health (Series)
Description: Baltimore : Johns Hopkins University Press, 2017. | Series:
    Operation health | Includes bibliographical references and index.
Identifiers: LCCN 2016025746 | ISBN 9781421422121 (pbk. : alk. paper) | ISBN
    1421422123 (pbk. : alk. paper) | ISBN 9781421422138 (electronic) | ISBN
    1421422131 (electronic)
Subjects: | MESH: Hemorrhagic Fever, Ebola—epidemiology | Surgical
    Procedures, Operative—standards | Disease Transmission,
    Infectious—prevention & control | Patient Care—ethics | Africa,
    Western—epidemiology | United States—epidemiology
Classification: LCC RC140.5 | NLM WC 534 | DDC 614.5/7—dc23
    LC record available at https://lccn.loc.gov/2016025746

A catalog record for this book is available from the British Library.

*Special discounts are available for bulk purchases of this book. For more information, please
contact Special Sales at 410-516-6936 or specialsales@press.jhu.edu.*

Johns Hopkins University Press uses environmentally friendly book materials,
including recycled text paper that is composed of at least 30 percent post-consumer
waste, whenever possible.

To T. T. Rodgers, Martin Salia, Samuel Batty, and Joseph Ngegba, and the many other healthcare workers who died during the West African Ebola outbreak

Contents

Contributors

Kathryn P. Barron, NP
Partners in Health
Boston, MA, USA

Håkon A. Bolkan, MD
Department of Cancer Research and Molecular Medicine
Norwegian University of Science and Technology
Trondheim, Norway

Séverine Caluwaerts, MD
Gynaecologist Technical Referent
Médecins Sans Frontières, Operating Center Brussels
Brussels, Belgium

Joseph Forrester, MD, MSc
Epidemic Intelligence Service Officer, Centers for Disease Control
Lieutenant, United States Public Health Service
Department of Surgery, Stanford University
Palo Alto, CA, USA

Andrew M. R. Hall, DipHE
Partners in Health
Boston, MA, USA

Eva Hanciles, MD, FWACS
Department of Anesthesiology
Princess Christian Maternity Hospital
Freetown, Sierra Leone

Mark J. Harris, MD, MPH
Department of Anesthesiology
University of Utah
Salt Lake City, UT, USA

Angela Hewlett, MD, MS
Assistant Professor, Division of Infectious Diseases
Associate Medical Director, Department of Infection Control and Epidemiology
Associate Medical Director, Nebraska Biocontainment Unit
Director, Infectious Diseases Outpatient Clinics
University of Nebraska Medical Center
Omaha, NE, USA

David B. Hoyt, MD, FACS
Executive Director
American College of Surgeons
Chicago, IL, USA

Daniel W. Johnson, MD
Division Chief, Critical Care
Department of Anesthesiology
University of Nebraska Medical Center
Omaha, NE, USA

Thaim B. Kamara, MBBS, FWACS
Department of Surgery
Connaught Hospital
Freetown, Sierra Leone

Songor S. J. Koedoyoma, MD
Koidu Government Hospital
Kono, Sierra Leone

Michael Koroma, MD, FWACS
Department of Anesthesiology
Princess Christian Maternity Hospital
Freetown, Sierra Leone

Adam L. Kushner, MD, MPH, FACS
Founder and Director, Surgeons OverSeas
New York, NY, USA
Lecturer, Department of Surgery, Columbia University
New York, NY, USA
Associate, Department of International Health
Johns Hopkins Bloomberg School of Public Health
Baltimore, MD, USA

Marta Lado, MD, DTMH
Clinical Lead
Kings Sierra Leone Partnership
Freetown, Sierra Leone

Ronald C. Marsh, MD, MIPH
Koidu Government Hospital
Kono, Sierra Leone

Andrew J. Michaels, MD, MPH, FACS
Partners in Health
Boston, MA, USA

Mohamed G. Sheku, MD
Koidu Government Hospital
Kono, Sierra Leone

Sherry M. Wren, MD, FACS, FCS(ECSA)
Professor of Surgery
Director of Global Surgery, Center for Global Health and
Innovation, Stanford University
Director, Clinical Surgery, Palo Alto Veterans Hospital
Palo Alto, CA, USA

Series Editor's Foreword

I know someone who needed surgery. He was born by emergent cesarean section. He had urgent stomach surgery at 2 months and an appendectomy at 23.

He is alive today because of surgery. I am that person.

Throughout much of the world, the lack of surgical care leads to death or disability for millions of men, women, and children. Yet despite this reality, the global health community has not fully recognized the urgent need for improving surgical care. Surgery and anesthesia are integral to the treatment of traumatic injuries and obstructed labor. Many infectious complications need surgery. Surgery is often the best or only treatment for many cancers. During conflict and after disasters, populations are vulnerable and need surgical care. But millions of people around the world lack access to such care.

I cannot say exactly what led me to train as a surgeon and practice in the developing world. What I do know is that to prepare to practice overseas, in the middle of my surgical training, I obtained a master of public health degree from Johns Hopkins University. At that time—1998—there was almost no mention of surgery within public health. I remember knocking on dozens of doors. I asked everyone about public health research projects that included surgical care. Time after time no one could help me.

I was not discouraged. I felt there must be a need for surgical care and so finished my surgery training. For a decade I practiced and taught in countries ranging from Iraq to Indonesia, Sierra Leone to South Sudan, and Niger to Nicaragua. My public health training had included a great deal about infectious diseases such as HIV, tuberculosis, and malaria. The reality that I began to see was that surgical care was also needed. I treated women in obstructed labor, children with appendicitis and typhoid perforations, and adults with fractures, hernias, and cancer. Many of these patients presented with late-stage disease. I began to wonder, How many patients were not seeking care? How many were dying in their villages and fields? How many were not as fortunate as I?

In 2008, along with local colleagues, I began documenting deficiencies in providing surgical care. A study in Sierra Leone showed no compressed oxygen, limited quantities of sterile gloves and eye protection, and only 10 surgeons for a population of 6 million. We showed that Sierra Leone hospitals in 2008 were worse off than US Civil War hospitals in 1864. Later, we conducted population-based surveys of surgical need in Sierra Leone, Rwanda, and Nepal. Estimates showed that up to 25% of the populations needed an operation and that access to surgery might have averted up to 33% of deaths. We had begun providing the evidence showing that millions of people around the world needed and wanted surgical care.

In 2013, I began teaching a course called "Surgical Care Needs in Low and Middle Income Countries" at the Johns Hopkins Bloomberg School of Public Health. The course covered surgical epidemiology, surgery for women and children, and surgical care during conflict and disasters. It was one of the first global surgery courses taught in the United States and the first at Johns Hopkins. Surgery and anesthesia had finally made a toehold in public health.

The course also led to Johns Hopkins University Press publishing *Operation Health: Surgical Care in the Developing World*. It was the first book in what would become the Operation Health series. The chapters begin with a personal vignette; then, experts from around the globe present case studies, best practices, and topic overviews. Chapters cover subjects such as cesarean sections in Ethiopia, clubfoot in Nepal, trauma in Tanzania, anesthesia in Ghana, and laparoscopy in Mongolia. The book is meant to speak to clinicians, students, and the general public. I hoped that it would educate and enlighten readers who would care about global surgery, many of whom just didn't yet know they cared.

With the success and interest generated by the first book, I developed a series covering the various aspects of the massive surgical needs in the developing world. Future books will cover conflict and disasters; cancer; women's health; child health; surgical subspecialties; and anesthesia and critical care. Following the blueprint of the first book, each volume will be short, suitable for students, clinicians, and the interested general public.

As the field of global surgery matures within global health, the question is not *should* we provide surgical care but *how*. By providing rich and accessible overviews alongside lessons learned from personal experiences, the Operation Health series begins to provide some ways forward.

Adam L. Kushner, MD, MPH, FACS

Foreword

This volume is an exciting contribution to our understanding not only of the disease Ebola but also of the need for a caring international response to a disease crisis. What have we learned from this as we go forward?

Our knowledge of Ebola is evolving, much as our knowledge about disaster preparedness in the United States evolved following the events of 9/11. What we know when an outbreak begins, though based on reliable sources, may not always be the final word. We look to governments and experts, other surgeons and professional societies, and we learn from resources on the Internet. We used all of these when dealing with the West African Ebola outbreak.

Nothing is a substitute for personal experience when complex problems need a response. All of these problems are further aggravated by a disease emerging in countries that are underdeveloped, lack material resources, have limited medical infrastructure, and limited finances. The Ebola outbreak was aggravated by a particularly high risk to healthcare workers and evolving information about appropriate personal protection when caring for infected patients.

The White House and US Department of State tried to establish international priorities. These priorities consisted of controlling the outbreak by helping to develop additional facilities to isolate and care for the patients, mitigating the economic instability by working with the International Monetary Fund, providing international coordination along with other countries and nongovernmental organizations, and developing policies to strengthen global security to try and prevent the spread outside of the outbreak area.

The International Incident Command Center was established in Monrovia, Liberia, for overall supervision, and efforts were developed in the United States through the combined efforts of the Centers for Disease Control and Prevention, Department of Health and Human Services, and Department of Defense to address epidemiology, infection and disease control, emergency medical services and hospital readiness, and treatment guidelines for personal protection.

These efforts led to some controversies about personal protection, but the American College of Surgeons, through the efforts of Drs. Wren, Kushner, and others, developed principles for personal protection for physicians and others performing surgery.

Now that Ebola is better controlled in West Africa and the threat of a worldwide epidemic seems to be past, it is essential to learn from this experience. The precise insights that the people caring for these patients share with us in these chapters will give us the basis to learn and develop and plan for any future outbreaks. Several things also emerge in reading about these experiences. First, we must acknowledge the incredible courage of our colleagues who put themselves at personal risk and provided care for those in need. This is the essence of professionalism in humanity. I am personally inspired by reading these stories, and they have reawakened my commitment to try and help in the future.

It is very important to create an international focus in helping countries when they face such problems. The awareness of the magnitude of surgical need globally is increasing, and Drs. Wren and Kushner's book describes opportunities for resource-rich countries to provide leadership, resources, and assistance to countries such as Sierra Leone, Liberia, and Guinea. We need to recommit our interest in humanity toward others around the world and allow development of medical infrastructure in countries to avoid this kind of crisis in the future.

David B. Hoyt, MD, FACS
Executive Director
American College of Surgeons

Preface

There are untold stories about death during the time of Ebola. These deaths resulted not just from Ebola virus disease (EVD) infections but also from medical and surgical conditions that were neglected. These non-EVD deaths were mostly not tallied and are not included in the total number reported of EVD deaths. These deaths were people who did not receive care for conditions resulting from injuries, obstructed labor, perforated stomach ulcers, or endemic infectious diseases such as malaria and tuberculosis. These secondary victims of EVD died because there were neither healthcare workers to provide care nor supplies to care for them safely. The aim of this book is to present the view from the United States and on the ground in West Africa, to highlight stories of surgical care and EVD. We aim to recount lessons learned and understand how we can better prepare for a future outbreak.

EVD, a viral hemorrhagic disease named for a 150-mile-long river in what is now the Democratic Republic of the Congo (DRC), first became known to the world in 1976, when 381 people in what was then called Zaire rapidly contracted the disease. An astounding 88% died horrible deaths. Since then the virus has surfaced multiple times but never infected more than 500 people in any specific outbreak.

On March 23, 2014, the African Regional Office of the World Health Organization (WHO) reported the first official cases of EVD in Guinea. Seven days later Liberia confirmed its first case. Within two months the disease had spread to Sierra Leone.

Nongovernmental organizations, ministries of health, and the US Centers for Disease Control and Prevention (CDC) started responding. What no one was prepared for was the intensity and intractability of the disease. On August 8, 2014, the WHO declared the outbreak a public health emergency of international concern. For people in the United States the outbreak was merely a news item, something US healthcare workers could volunteer to travel to Africa to help with or a theoretical exercise in US hospital responsiveness.

That changed on September 30, 2014, when Thomas Eric Duncan, a Liberian national, presented to a Texas hospital and eventually was diagnosed with EVD. Within two weeks he was dead and two healthcare workers in the hospital also contracted the disease. The US political and media frenzy that followed disseminated fear and misinformation and led to widespread discrimination of anything "African." US hospitals scrambled to make sure they were EVD-ready and personal protective equipment (PPE) was stockpiled.

In the end, while almost 18,000 people in the United States had laboratory-confirmed cases of influenza, only four were diagnosed with EVD: the three from Texas and one New York physician who turned EVD positive after returning from volunteering in West Africa. The impact in West Africa, however, was much worse, with nearly 30,000 infected with EVD and more than 17,000 EVD deaths. Also of significance was the decimation of healthcare workers in countries that already had insufficient workforces for their populations.

This book, part of the Johns Hopkins University Press series on surgical care in the developing world, is a collection of healthcare workers' stories on surgical care during the 2014-2015 West African EVD outbreak. The book is divided into three sections: the view from the United States, the view from Sierra Leone, and technical considerations and the way forward. In Part I, Chapter 1 recognizes the need for and development of an Ebola and surgery guideline. Chapter 2 covers the Nebraska Biocontainment Unit and the care that was provided there. In Part II, Chapter 3 describes the personal thoughts and recollections behind the difficult decision to temporarily close the Médecins Sans Frontières maternity hospital. Chapter 4 is a chronology of the outbreak and treatment of EVD and non-EVD patients in Sierra Leone told from the perspective of the hospital care manager at Connaught Hospital. Chapter 5 looks at anesthesia and EVD. Chapter 6 looks at the decreased numbers of operations and the effects of EVD on a CapaCare Surgical Training Program.

Part III provides insights into successful programs and projects and provides evidence that surgical care is possible in a time of EVD. Chapter 7 describes the development of a maternity isolation unit at the Princess Christian Maternity Hospital in Freetown, Sierra Leone, and Chapter 8 highlights how surgery is done in a time of EVD. Chapter 9 looks at operating in personal protective equipment and gives best practices for how to do so safely. Chapter 10 is by a CDC Epidemic Information Service officer who also is a surgical resident. His account of gathering information in Liberia provides insights into how to monitor and evaluate an outbreak.

The individual chapters describe what occurred during the current outbreak, but they also provide suggestions and recommendations that will hopefully better prepare us for a future infectious disease outbreak. What initially was an isolated and remote problem quickly became one that affected all nations of the world. Fortunately, despite the initial despair, there was a glimmer of hope.

Timeline

2013

December 6   Death of "patient zero," a 2-year-old boy in Guinea.

2014

March 23   Ministry of Health of Guinea notified World Health Organization of Ebola outbreak.

March 27   First confirmed cases in Conakry, Guinea.

March 30   First confirmed cases in Liberia.

May 26   First confirmed cases in Sierra Leone.

June 17   First confirmed cases in Monrovia, Liberia.

June 28   First confirmed case in Freetown, Sierra Leone.

July 29   Dr. Sheik Umar Khan first healthcare worker to die in Sierra Leone.

August 2   Dr. Kent Brantly infected in Liberia and evacuated for treatment at Emory University.

September 4   Rick Sacra infected in Liberia and evacuated to Nebraska Medical Center.

September 30   Centers for Disease Control and Prevention confirmed first case in Americas of Thomas Eric Duncan in Dallas, Texas.

October 16   Médecins Sans Frontières announced closure of Gondama Referral Center in Sierra Leone.

November 15   Dr. Martin Salia, a surgeon working in Sierra Leone, was evacuated to Nebraska.

November 17   Dr. Salia died.

2015

May 1   WHO declared cases exceed 26,300, with 10,900 deaths.

May 9   Liberia declared Ebola-free.

June 29   New cases detected in Liberia.

September 3   Liberia declared Ebola-free.

November 7   Sierra Leone declared Ebola-free.

2016

January 14   WHO declared end of West African Ebola outbreak,
                with over 11,300 deaths. Later that day, confirmed case
                reported in Sierra Leone.

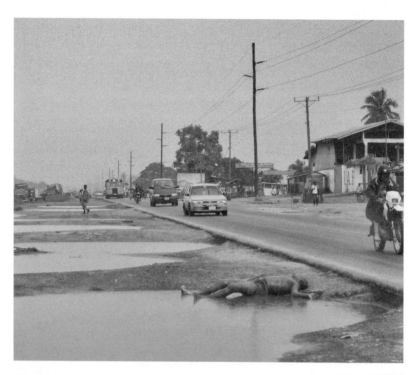

Abandoned body, Monrovia, Liberia. July 2014.
Photo courtesy Joseph Forrester

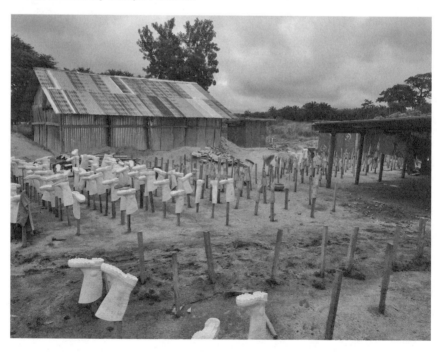

Boots drying in Liberia. Photo courtesy Joseph Forrester

Operation Ebola

| THE VIEW FROM THE UNITED STATES

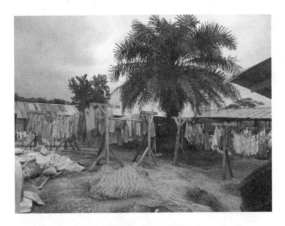

Clothes washing station, Ebola Treatment Unit,
Northern Liberia. Photo courtesy Joseph Forrester

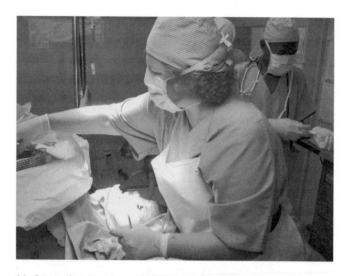

1.1. Operating in a low-resource environment. Photo courtesy
Sherry M. Wren

1

Filling the Void

Drafting Guidelines for Surgery and Ebola

SHERRY M. WREN, MD, FACS, FCS(ECSA),

AND ADAM L. KUSHNER, MD, MPH, FACS

In August and September 2014, global media outlets were beginning to talk more about the unfolding Ebola crisis in Africa. For us, this was not really news; we had closely followed the progress of Ebola virus disease (EVD) from isolated cases in Guinea, to the mass quarantines in Liberia, and the deaths in Freetown, Sierra Leone. We both had worked as surgeons in the region and had friends there. Discussions started between us about the conditions our African colleagues were working in and how they could remain safe but still deliver important care.

For Sherry this was a bit of a flashback, as she had started her surgical residency in 1986 at Yale New Haven Hospital during the height of AIDS as an untreatable lethal disease. Infected patients had yellow charts so everyone knew they had AIDS, and surgery was commonly being performed to diagnose and treat some of the AIDS-related problems. Then in August 1988 a medical resident became acutely infected with HIV after a needle stick injury, and the media storm in the hospital lobby about letting the AIDS-infected doctor work left an indelible memory.

It is hard to believe that there was no "Universal Precautions" policy and that surgeons, doctors, nurses, and hospital staff wore no gloves or other personal protective gear while handling possibly infected bodily fluids at that time. In June 1988 the Centers for Disease Control and Prevention (CDC) came out with the first guidelines to try and protect healthcare workers from hepatitis and HIV infection, but it took years for this to become standard practice in every hospital. Fast-forward to 2014, and the parallels of the EVD outbreak to AIDS are glaringly obvious.

Since both of us had operated extensively in African countries, we were aware of the existing inadequacies of personal protective equipment (PPE) prior to this outbreak. Typical African operating room attire is cotton scrubs with a plastic butcher's apron over them to protect the chest and abdomen from blood soaking through. Over this is a cotton gown that is not a fluid barrier and allows blood and fluid to contact the surgical staffs' skin on the arms, necks, legs, or anywhere there is no plastic apron. This is vastly different from attire in a typical US operating room, where a fluid barrier gown, eye protection, and impervious patient drapes are standard for every case.

Knowing the probable deficiencies, Adam contacted Dr. Thaim B. Kamara, a longtime friend and colleague who was also a surgeon and hospital care manager at Connaught Hospital in Freetown, Sierra Leone, to ask what was happening. The response was chilling. The description would upset any surgeon. Patients were denied care because of suspected EVD infections. Many patients were dying. The surgeons were indeed operating, but the number of cases had drastically decreased and there was a lack of protective items and supplies. (For more details see Chapter 4.)

Immediately we thought to try and help. Surgeons OverSeas (SOS), a nongovernmental organization based in the United States that had worked at Connaught Hospital, wired some funds to purchase cleaning material locally, but this was not enough. Soon, however, there was a worldwide outcry and personnel and supplies to the area began to arrive.

The other thing we realized was that there were no guidelines or protocols on caring for a surgical patient with suspected or confirmed EVD. What if there was a case in the United States? What if our colleagues or we needed to operate? How were our friends and colleagues in West Africa going to remain safe and able to help in their hospitals? Infectious disease and public health experts were asked about surgery and EVD and universally replied, "Why would anyone think of worrying about that?" The lack of understanding that patients would still need access to procedures when they may have Ebola was on no one's mind.

To help guide colleagues in West Africa living with this question, we searched the medical literature, the World Health Organization (WHO), and the CDC websites for PPE guidelines for EVD and surgery or invasive procedures. There was a guideline on how and when to breast-feed with

EVD but nothing about how to operate and when. This absence of formal guidelines, which still exists at the time of writing this book, demonstrates what we believe is the lack of the public health community's understanding of the role surgical care plays in any crisis. In the end we decided that someone needed to correct this glaring omission, and so over the course of an evening, we sent scores of emails back and forth between Palo Alto and Baltimore and devised a draft of the "Ebola and Surgery guideline."

Within a few hours we learned what we could about Association for the Advancement of Medical Instrumentation (AMMI) gown and drape standards for virus and blood imperviousness and reviewed existing PPE guidelines. Operating room instruments and sharps management were then added, as were protocols for operating on known blood-borne diseases. The draft was certainly not perfect, but it was a start and was intended as a provocation to encourage entities such as the WHO and the CDC to write definitive guideline with their imprimatur.

We sent the draft to David B. Hoyt, MD, FACS, executive director of the American College of Surgeons (ACS) for review and endorsement. Dr. Hoyt, as a trauma and disaster response expert, recognized the need and the void, approved the draft, and made sure it was forwarded to the nearly 80,000 US and international ACS members. The next morning it was featured on the ACS website. The draft guidelines were also forwarded to the leaders of other professional societies and organizations in the United States and throughout Africa. By the end of the week, nearly a dozen groups had endorsed the guidelines.

The guidelines themselves were broken down into recommendations about patient selection, PPE, conduct of the procedure, checklist, and specimen handling. The patient selection recommendations were soon revised as more information became available. They currently state:

Elective surgical procedures should not be performed in cases of suspected or confirmed Ebola (EVD). Emergency operations can be considered in cases as defined by the CDC: Persons Under Investigation, Probable Cases, and early Confirmed Cases. Patients with severe active disease would not likely tolerate an operation due to the severity of their disease. Any decision to operate should weigh all risks and benefits; specifically the risk of death from the current severity of their EVD, risk of death from their surgical disease, and risk of exposure to the operating room team against the likelihood of potential benefit of emergency surgery. Choice of operative approach (open or minimally invasive) should take into consideration minimizing potential hazards to all members of the operating room team.

The response by surgical colleagues in Africa was heartening; the College of Surgeons of East, Central, and South Africa, a ten-country consortium, rapidly adopted and transmitted the document throughout its membership. In March 2015 Sherry, Thaim Kamara from Sierra Leone, and Dr. Lawrence Sherman from Liberia addressed the West African College of Surgeons, a consortium of 26 Francophone and Anglophone countries about EVD and its effect on surgical care.

The public health community has been slow to recognize the importance of surgical care. But this EVD outbreak has given us a glimpse of a world without it. Even in the United States, injured patients in need of surgery who returned from EVD-affected countries—despite testing negative for the disease—were forced to wait 21 days before a US surgeon would operate.

The EVD outbreak in West Africa seems to have abated and a global crisis averted, for now. We believe that now is the time to discuss and plan for what happens when the next infectious disease outbreak confronts us. Are we not morally obligated to provide surgical care to those in need but also to ensure that healthcare workers throughout the world have access to PPE to minimize their risk of contracting the disease from the patients they are treating? In this crisis nearly 900 healthcare workers in West Africa were infected with EVD. Over 500 died. This is in a setting where the number of healthcare workers to treat the populations of the three countries is already grossly inadequate.

Santayana wrote in 1905, "Those who cannot remember the past are condemned to repeat it." Our worry is unless something changes we are going to repeat the same issues: first AIDS, then SARS, EVD, MERS, and whatever challenge comes next. The time to invest in health infrastructure, including surgical care (surgery, anesthesia, obstetrics, and nursing), is now.

ADDITIONAL READING

Crompton J, Kingham TP, Kamara TB, Brennan MF, Kushner AL. Comparison of surgical care deficiencies between US civil war hospitals and present-day hospitals in Sierra Leone. *World J Surg*. 2010 Aug;34(8):1743-7.

Sherman L, Clement PT, Cherian MN, Ndayimirije N, Noel L, Dahn B, Gwenigale WT, Kushner AL. Implementing Liberia's poverty reduction strategy: an assessment of emergency and essential surgical care. *Arch Surg.* 2011 Jan;146(1):35-9.

Wren SM, Kushner AL. Surgical protocol for possible or confirmed Ebola cases, *https://www.facs.org/surgeons/ebola/surgical-protocol* (accessed February 15, 2016).

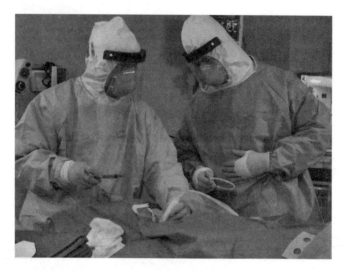

2.1. Placement of a central venous catheter in the Nebraska Biocontainment Unit. Photo courtesy Kathleen C. Boulter

2

The United States' Domestic

Response to Ebola

Experience of the Nebraska

Biocontainment Unit

ANGELA HEWLETT, MD, MS, AND DANIEL W. JOHNSON, MD

The Nebraska Biocontainment Unit (NBU) was designed to care for patients with highly infectious diseases while protecting healthcare workers, a need brought to the forefront in 2003, when many healthcare workers became ill while treating patients with SARS. The concept of a biocontainment patient care unit was nothing new; however, there were only a few in the United States. Since there were no national standards for these units, experts from existing units assembled and published a consensus statement in 2006 detailing their design, planning, and operations. In spite of this guidance, biocontainment patient care units remained a rarity in the United States, mostly due to funding constraints.

From 2005 to 2014, the NBU remained ready to receive patients with highly infectious diseases; however, this did not occur. Often I (AH) was asked, "What did you do for nine years if you had no patients?" My response was that we were quite busy in spite of not having an active patient in the NBU. We planned and executed quarterly drills with the entire healthcare team, performed multiple research projects on appropriate personal protective equipment (PPE) use, decontamination, and modeling of pathogen trajectory, and led a significant amount of education of healthcare workers and first responders in the community. Was the NBU a part of my job? Certainly. Was it the main component of my job? Definitely not. This changed dramatically in 2014.

I distinctly remember receiving a call in early August 2014 from the medical director of the NBU, Dr. Phil Smith. The US Department of State had requested to visit the NBU to assess our capabilities in the midst of

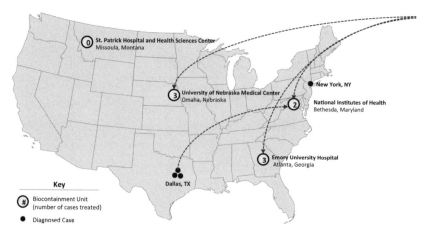

2.2. Map of the United States—biocontainment units and diagnosed cases. Courtesy G. Taylor Corbett

the escalating outbreak of Ebola virus disease (EVD) in West Africa. We were following the outbreak closely, as we had with previous outbreaks of various infectious diseases throughout the world. We knew immediately that EVD presented the potential for opening the NBU for the first time. We assumed that the scenario would involve an ill traveler presenting to an ER somewhere in the United States and being transported to us; however, the arrival of the first two patients with EVD to the Serious Communicable Diseases Unit at Emory University signaled that this was indeed different, since these patients were healthcare workers who had been medically evacuated from Africa.

Needing additional facilities for EVD patients in the United States, the Department of State representatives traveled around the country and visited several facilities to assess capabilities. They deemed the NBU equipped and ready to care for an EVD patient. We received the call from the Department of State in early September, informing us that our first patient with EVD would arrive on September 5, 2014. Our team shifted into high gear. I remember this intense preparation process and how it was so gratifying to watch our team come together for the actual instead of the theoretical. None of our team members backed away when they received the activation call. Instead they stood ready when our patient arrived; they were anxious for what the day would bring yet excited to have the opportunity to care for someone who needed us.

Our preparation escalated as we readied the NBU to receive our patient. We prepared our existing team of nurses, physicians, and others, and notified additional physicians (Critical Care Medicine, Anesthesiology) that we would likely need their services. We answered many questions along the way to ensure that our assembled team was willing and able to provide care to a patient with EVD. There was some discussion regarding the ethical obligation of physicians to provide care for patients with EVD. In actuality we wanted only those who were engaged and willing to provide care in the NBU to streamline the process and decrease anxiety as much as possible to ensure a safe environment. PPE, transport, and patient care protocols were meticulously reviewed and revised specifically for EVD, and supplies were gathered.

Reality of Providing Care

On September 4, 2014, I (DJ) received a phone call from the director of critical care at the University of Nebraska Medical Center (UNMC): "Dan, did you know that we have a patient with Ebola coming from Liberia tomorrow?" This was a question that I did not expect to hear during my entire career as an anesthesiologist and intensivist. While the situation seemed surreal, I knew that it was time to get mentally prepared to face this deadly disease head on.

I learned that our first patient was a physician. I immediately Googled him and read about his work in Liberia and how he chose to continue in his healthcare mission despite the risk of contracting EVD. While I tried to remain nonemotional and objective about our medical plan for him, I couldn't help but feel that this brave physician-brother of ours deserved an extraordinary effort to help him survive. After all, he had put his own life on the line for strangers with EVD.

The handoff reports I received during the transportation from Liberia were fairly spotty. We knew that he was awake, he was breathing on his own, and that his vital signs were nearly normal. The transport plane landed in Omaha about 6:00 a.m. I went upstairs to the NBU to await his arrival.

While it seems hard to believe now, back on September 5, 2014, I barely knew any of the NBU physicians, nurses, and staff. We intensivists had only recently become involved with the drills and preparations for EVD. That first morning, I was struck by the mood of my colleagues in the NBU. They appeared focused, concerned, under stress but not at all overwhelmed. The entire staff appeared to be of the same mindset: we have prepared for this challenge and we can succeed in the care of this patient. While I felt somewhat awkward introducing myself to so many NBU workers on such a monumental day, I was given a warm welcome. This helped me to manage my own apprehension about the situation.

The leaders of the NBU really rose to the occasion. Drs. Smith and Hewlett (NBU medical directors), Shelly Schwedhelm (nursing director), Kate Boulter (lead nurse), Dr. Shawn Gibbs (decontamination specialist), and Dr. John Lowe (transport specialist) answered every question we had. While I had good reason to be fearful of the hours to come, I took comfort in the firm confidence I saw in their eyes.

When I saw our patient wheeled past me in his plastic suit, I thought, "Is there any way we can get him to survive?" While we *now* know that EVD is survivable, in September 2014, most Americans (including myself) still regarded it as unsurvivable. As an intensivist, I care for patients with overwhelming sepsis on a regular basis. Regardless of how deranged their vital signs are, I almost never question whether I can help them survive—I assume that I can restore them to health. With EVD, the feeling was different. Despite his nearly normal vital signs, I felt like the deck was stacked against him.

Following the initial assessment of our patient, I collaborated with the Infectious Disease doctors to make a treatment plan. A central venous catheter (a large intravenous line typically placed in the jugular vein in the neck) was needed. In the 30 minutes leading up to that first invasive procedure, I felt a wave of conflicting emotions. I was confident that I would successfully and safely place the central line, as I had placed so many in the last 10 years. But my mind wandered to my wife, my daughter, and my son. I couldn't help but fear the sadness I would put on my dear family if I made an error and had a needle stick exposure to EVD. Kate Boulter and Dr. Angela Hewlett helped me don PPE for the procedure. They asked me if I felt safe and confident in the PPE, and I surely did. As I started to walk toward our patient's room, I took a pause as I thought of my wife and kids. I felt an anxiety that I had not felt in many years. I knew that I needed to perform at a very high level and that these thoughts were a barrier to optimal care.

I psyched myself up by thinking of military personnel, police officers, and firefighters. These brave people receive specialized training and equipment, and when duty calls they put fear aside and they do the job that needs to be done. I, too, had received specialized training, I had all of the equipment I needed, and I knew that I could safely place that line. I said an "Our Father" followed by a "Hail Mary," as I have done thousands of times throughout my life. I asked God to protect me and to bless my hands. Then I walked through the door.

Once I was able to see our patient with my own eyes, my fears went away. What I saw was a human being who needed my help. I told him that his work in Liberia was heroic and that we would do everything in our power to restore him to health. He was fairly somnolent at that time, but I think he nodded to express some degree of understanding. I then placed the central line without incident. Performing invasive procedures while in full PPE is not the same as performing them under normal circumstances. Over the course of the outbreak, I placed three central venous catheters in patients' jugular veins, one arterial catheter in the wrist, and one breathing tube in the trachea. Each of these procedures could be put into one of two categories. When they went swiftly and smoothly, I hardly noticed or cared that I was wearing full PPE. When they were challenging and took longer than 30 minutes, the presence of the PPE became a real problem, mainly because of the heat. During any stressful procedure, body heat and sweating increase, and when the body heat and sweat are trapped inside your suit, the problem compounds itself. I can imagine the physical challenge of providing care in the summer heat of West Africa, considering the experience of doing this in an air-conditioned US hospital. At the conclusion of each one of my invasive procedures, I felt tremendous relief and I was so happy that I had been able to contribute to the care of our patient.

Donning PPE took approximately 10 minutes, which is significantly longer than the normal amount of time necessary to don regular surgical attire. The main reasons for the difference are the double-checking that we do (to ensure zero possible breaches) and the duct-taping of gloves to gown (to ensure fluid tight seals). Doffing PPE took approximately 10 to 15 minutes, and it followed a meticulous list of instructions created and constantly evaluated by the NBU staff. To avoid self-contamination, I listened more carefully to my doffing partner than I have ever listened to anyone before or since. In short, I did exactly as I was told, and I made no sudden movements.

After three weeks of treatment in the NBU, our first patient walked out of UNMC looking tired but healthy. He had recovered from EVD, and our campus felt joy and pride the likes of which I have never seen before. Having a conversation with our patient without wearing PPE, along with his wife and children, was one of the true highlights of my career.

While I had very little involvement with the second patient in the NBU, my experience with EVD was far from over. In November 2014 I had the privilege and honor of caring for our third patient. He was a US national who had been working as a general surgeon at Connaught Hospital in his native Sierra Leone when he contracted EVD. (For more detail see Chapter 4.) His initial testing may have been early enough in the course to yield a false negative. His subsequent course and testing confirmed that he was suffering from EVD.

Within an hour of his arrival in the NBU, we knew that he had an extremely small chance of survival. I remember looking at Dr. Hewlett's face after we received the results on his initial metabolic laboratory tests; we mirrored each other's grave concerns. EVD had clearly ravaged multiple organ systems, and we feared that we had received him in the NBU a few days too late.

Dr. Smith and I met with our patient's wife as soon as she arrived in Omaha. We explained that his condition was extremely critical and that we would try our best to reverse the course of his disease. She expressed understanding and she described the intense faith in God that she and her husband had developed together. It was his faith that had guided him to care for the people of Sierra Leone.

Our team tried everything. We placed a central line, an arterial line, a hemodialysis catheter, and an endotracheal tube. We performed X-rays, echocardiograms, ultrasounds, and every laboratory test available. We provided fluids, electrolytes, convalescent plasma, blood, ZMapp, vasopressors, inotropes, continuous dialysis, and mechanical ventilation. We used expertise from more than 15 physicians on-site and dozens more from other campuses via telephone and email. With every set of results we obtained, we could see that we were fighting a disease that refused to relinquish control of his body.

When our patient went into cardiac arrest, I was at his side. When it became clear that our efforts were futile, I directed the team to stop. We all felt a tremendous sadness. I held his hand and thought about what an incredible loss his family and West Africa had just sustained. I felt guilty for failing to keep him alive, yet I felt privileged that I had the opportunity to care for such an altruistic man.

The weeks following the death of our patient were perhaps the most difficult weeks of my career. While I received supportive words from many people, my mind continued to analyze every decision we had made, searching for some theoretical pathway that could have resulted in survival.

During the 21-day period of temperature monitoring that most experts agree is the incubation period for EVD, my 3-year-old daughter developed a high fever without any other symptoms. Although the rational part of my brain *knew* that it was impossible for me to transmit EVD without having any signs of the disease myself, the emotional part of my brain was overwhelmed by the thought that I had given the disease to my beautiful little girl. I called Dr. Hewlett daily to receive reassurance that my daughter could not possibly have EVD. The fever lasted for five days, including Thanksgiving. I placed myself in a sort of pseudoquarantine that week, working until late in the evening at my office and sleeping at my parents' house to avoid any contact with my wife and children. I skipped our large family Thanksgiving feast because I didn't want any of my aunts, uncles, or cousins to feel stress from being near an Ebola healthcare provider. After a week of being isolated from each other, my wife and children and I rejoiced when my daughter's fever subsided and we were all together again.

My wife endured tremendous stress during the Ebola outbreak. While all spouses of critical care physicians have to deal with difficult schedules and unpredictable hours, most do not have to wonder, as my wife did, "Will my husband be exposed to Ebola today? Is there any way that he might transmit the disease to our children? What would life be like if he died as a result of this work?" For the most part, she kept these emotions bottled up and only expressed her support and pride at our efforts. She also provided extensive emotional support to me following the devastating loss of our third patient. I felt a lot of personal responsibility and guilt in the months that followed, and she was able to steer me back on track by reminding me that we had given him the very best chance at survival. All family members of healthcare workers in contact with Ebola dealt with challenges, and in a way, they were the unsung heroes of the entire ordeal.

Lessons Learned

Our experiences in the NBU taught us many lessons, which we carry with us as we see patients in other areas of the hospital. Trust meant everything in the NBU. Our donning and doffing partners became our best friends, since we knew they were protecting us from exposure. Practicing donning and doffing of PPE was important, but the presence of a trained observer was the most helpful part of this process. Our team was responsible for all of the activities inside the NBU, including all cleaning tasks. Although these tasks may not fit a usual job description, it was understood that this was an important part of preventing unnecessary exposures and enhancing safety. We trusted our fellow team members to perform these tasks in a complete and safe manner.

We learned not to resist change. It is important to have preexisting protocols in place, but it was more important to keep these fluid. The NBU had many existing protocols, and we were thankful for these guidance documents. We did, however, modify them on an ongoing basis, and continue to do so. If a better way to do something was discovered with experience, we made changes as necessary. We learned to listen to the nurses at the bedside. They constantly made improvements to existing protocols, sometimes finding novel ways to make a process safer or find optimal patient care equipment. The NBU team held a daily meeting called "the huddle" during activation. This enabled any team member to voice an opinion on potential improvements and to influence change in policy.

EVD patients generate a large amount of waste, which must be disposed of in a safe manner. We were fortunate to have an autoclave installed in the NBU, which saved us from arranging for disposal of waste through an outside vendor (an incredibly difficult and expensive process). Everything that left the NBU passed through the autoclave first. One patient with EVD required constant operation of the autoclave for about 12 hours per day, so we found it necessary to provide a dedicated staff member to perform this task.

The ability to process laboratory specimens required a significant amount of consideration and input from multiple individuals. Prior to activation, our physician team generated a wish list of lab studies that we needed to care for a patient with EVD. Our laboratory director and staff evaluated this list and determined how to safely process the specimens. We learned to be receptive to the fact that unlike in a normal hospital setting, we cannot always draw every lab that we want at any time of day. By working closely with our laboratory, we were able to obtain a suitable list of lab studies we felt were necessary to care for our patients while maintaining the highest safety standards for our laboratory personnel.

Patients with EVD may recover clinically but still have detectable viral loads for a prolonged period of time. In a normal hospital environment patients who are feeling better are allowed to leave their room and walk in the hallways, meet with family members, and so on. In the NBU the patients must remain in their rooms until they meet discharge criteria as defined by the Centers for Disease Control and Prevention (CDC). Therefore, it was necessary to provide entertainment for patients. This included videoconferencing with family and friends, Internet and movie access, videoconferencing with physical therapy services, and an exercise bicycle in the patient room. One of our patients had a small basketball hoop and played chess with the nursing staff. NBU staff members brought in specially requested foods and engaged our patients in multiple activities throughout the day to combat boredom and feelings of isolation that are inherent to the biocontainment unit.

The administrative portion of caring for a patient with EVD required a significant amount of time. We participated in conference calls with various individuals and groups (CDC, World Health Organization, other academic centers, etc.) multiple times per day while caring for our patients. The media scrutiny was intense. It was imperative to have a public information officer (PIO) to actively participate as a member of the team and coordinate media requests. We found that it was extremely difficult to continue our "day jobs" in clinic, inpatient service, and so on while caring for a patient in the NBU. We required a significant amount of support from our practice partners to continue providing care for other patients while the NBU was activated. We also learned the importance of the extensive support we received from our UNMC hospital administration. Before, during, and after our activation, our colleagues and administrators at Nebraska Medicine rallied around our team and encouraged our efforts. Understandably, some people in the community questioned the use of resources devoted to such a small number of patients, but there was also a significant amount of pride in the NBU felt by both employees of Nebraska Medicine and residents of our community, who understood that we were not simply devoting enormous resources to promote the survival of three patients but were also aiding in the global response by learning how to safely and effectively care for patients with EVD.

This experience taught us to work as a true team. The unfortunate hierarchy system that is omnipresent on the wards does not apply in the NBU. Doctors, nurses, respiratory therapists, and others worked together to provide the best care for our patients while keeping each other safe. If someone pointed out a flaw in PPE or process, the culture of the NBU does not allow for defensiveness. Instead, you thank your colleague for the input and possibly for saving your life that day. When we see our fellow team members in the hallways of the hospital, we always stop and say hello and sometimes exchange stories of our time in the NBU. As a team we rejoiced together when our patients were doing well, and we cried together when our third patient died. Our time in the NBU was unlike any patient care experience in our careers.

Future Directions

It was a true privilege to provide care to our patients, who had given so much of themselves to help others. One of the best parts about being a healthcare worker is seeing a sick patient recover, and it was truly rewarding to see our first two EVD patients return home to their families and eventually return to Africa to continue their amazing work. Our feeling of elation on discharge day for our first two patients was absolutely indescribable, as was the crushing sorrow when we could not save the life of our third patient with EVD. The events of those days are permanently etched in our memory and will continue to resonate in our minds as we continue our work in the NBU. We feel that the true heroes of the EVD outbreak are the humanitarians who willingly left the safety of their home countries to help on the front lines, and we want to convey our heartfelt admiration for their altruism and courage. They are incredibly inspiring to us and to the other American and European healthcare providers who cared for patients with EVD outside of Africa. We went to work with all of the resources of modern, well-funded medical centers; they went to work in an extremely challenging environment without many of the supplies and resources they wanted and needed. Their accomplishments are simply amazing, and we sincerely thank them for their service.

Currently the NBU is working to educate other healthcare facilities on biocontainment and the safe care of patients with highly infectious diseases. We have been very open and transparent about sharing our protocols and procedures via the Internet and other outlets, and our team has been actively writing and publishing in the academic literature. The NBU was also selected to collaborate with Emory University, Bellevue Hospital Center, the Office of the Assistant Secretary for Preparedness and Response (ASPR), and the CDC to form the National Ebola Training and Education Center. We feel that the education of others is a good role for the NBU team, and we hope that our experience will translate into enhanced preparedness of other hospitals for EVD or other highly infectious diseases. After all, in an era of global travel dangerous infectious diseases are only a plane ride away.

ADDITIONAL READING

Hewlett AL, Varkey J, Smith PW, Ribner BS. Ebola virus disease: preparedness and infection control lessons learned from two biocontainment units. *Curr Opin Infect Dis.* 2015.28(4):343-348.

Johnson DW, Sullivan JN, Piquette CA, Hewlett AL, Bailey KL, Smith PW, Kalil AC, Lisco SJ. Lessons learned: critical care management of patients with Ebola in the United States. *Crit Care Med.* 2015 Jun;43(6):1157-64. doi: 10.1097/CCM.00000 00000000935.

Sueblinvong V, Johnson DW, Weinstein GL, Connor MJ Jr, Crozier I, Liddell AM, Franch HA, Wall BR, Kalil AC, Feldman M, Lisco SJ, Sevransky JE. Critical care for multiple organ failure secondary to Ebola virus disease in the United States. *Crit Care Med.* 2015 Oct;43(10):2066-75.

Uyeki TM, Mehta AK, Davey RT, et al. Clinical management of Ebola virus disease in the United States and Europe. *N Engl J Med.* 2016; 374:636-646

II THE VIEW FROM SIERRA LEONE

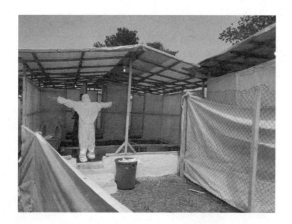

Disinfecting a worker at an Ebola Treatment
Unit, Monrovia, Liberia. Photo courtesy Joseph
Forrester

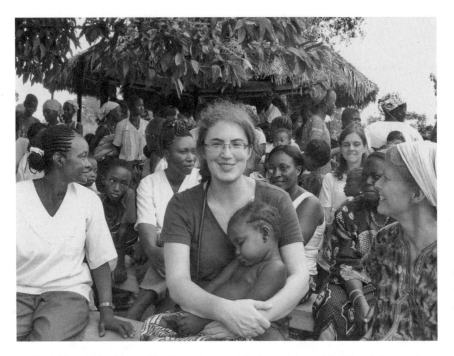

3.1. A friendship formed in Sierra Leone. Photo courtesy Séverine Caluwaerts

3

Closing the Médecins Sans Frontières

Maternity Hospital in Sierra Leone

SÉVERINE CALUWAERTS, MD

I am an obstetrician-gynecologist with Médecins Sans Frontières (MSF). Since 2008 I did five missions at the Gondama Referral Center (GRC) in Bo Province in central Sierra Leone. The hospital, a 200-bed facility, admitted children under 15 and women in need of obstetric and gynecologic care. MSF began providing pediatric care at GRC in 2003 and expanded to maternity cases in 2008. The facility was very busy, with over 8,000 pediatric and 2,500 obstetrical and gynecological admissions annually.

According to the World Health Organization, even before the Ebola virus disease (EVD) outbreak, Sierra Leone had the highest maternal mortality in the world. The lifetime risk of a woman dying of pregnancy-related complications in Sierra Leone was 1 in 21. At GRC, we lost on average 3 to 4 mothers a month due to bleeding, infection, or high blood pressure–related complications of pregnancy. The mothers I lost are etched on my soul. I remember their faces. I remember my feelings of inadequacy, anger, and sadness related to these maternal deaths. These mothers did not have to die. They died because the roads were bad; because transport was nonexistent; because they were referred too late; or because they did not receive the correct drugs before referral. Such were the baseline conditions in Sierra Leone before EVD.

My return to GRC in May 2014 coincided with the first EVD case crossing the border from Guinea to Sierra Leone. The virus knew no borders, and day by day we saw it approaching GRC. MSF had years of experience with EVD, and so we prepared as other MSF teams were treating patients in Guinea, Liberia, and throughout Sierra Leone. Though we hoped it would

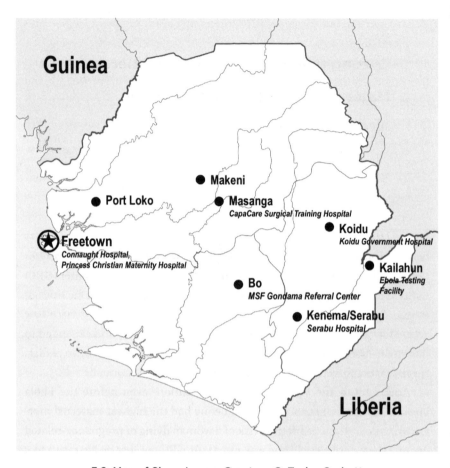

3.2. Map of Sierra Leone. Courtesy G. Taylor Corbett

not happen, each of us knew in our hearts that eventually EVD would reach Bo and GRC.

In July it did.

A pregnant woman with a very strong suspicion of EVD presented at our door. Our triage system functioned as it was supposed to, and she was screened and identified at the hospital entrance. She was placed in the isolation tent and treated there. She died a few days later. More cases followed. The staff was scared. I was scared.

EVD in a general hospital is devastating. Managing a large facility in full personal protective equipment (PPE) is almost impossible. MSF had strict policies and only allowed a maximum of three hours a day in full

PPE per person. But with 20 sick children and 10 sick pregnant women presenting daily, this was problematic. Many of our patients, since we were a referral hospital, fell under the case definition of EVD, with bleeding and fever. These are typical signs of EVD but also common with pregnancy and obstetric complications. We felt we could not offer quality care to patients presenting with these symptoms for fear of them having EVD. The blood, the amniotic fluid, the breast milk, all body fluids can be infected with the potentially deadly disease.

We did not want to abandon our patients, so we looked into different strategies to continue to provide care. One option was to test everyone before entering the facility and to let only EVD-negative women remain. It was an attractive idea but unrealistic. EVD test results took 24 hours because the samples needed to be sent to Kailahun. That meant, for example, a woman with heavy bleeding from placenta previa, with her baby in distress—an extreme emergency—remaining in front of the hospital for 24 hours while awaiting her test results. As humanitarians we could not watch women die waiting for tests, which might even be negative, while we might have had the means to save them.

Another option was to admit only two or three patients a day and manage them in full PPE with the staff we had. But this would mean that, if an ambulance arrived with two patients but we only had space for one, we could only admit one. We would need to "play God." Some patients would be cared for; others would not. Deciding who got the chance to live and who would probably die seemed inhuman.

A third option was to manage the maternity as an EVD treatment unit. It would mean all the staff working in full PPE and every patient considered EVD-positive until proven otherwise. We would have the difficult decision of operating on patients while awaiting their test results.

Previously I had operated on known hepatitis C and HIV-positive patients and patients with suspected Lassa Fever, an infectious disease also endemic in Sierra Leone. For those patients, I knew the risk of doing surgery. It was never zero, but it seemed acceptable. I was willing to accept the risk to save a patient's life. But with EVD the risks seemed too high. We were afraid that even a single needle stick injury from an EVD-positive patient might transmit the disease. I felt that we could not ask the national staff or the international staff to take such a life-threatening risk.

And having everyone work all the time in full PPE? Aside from the supply problem, this would mean needing to double our staff. We just did not have the capacity. So many MSF resources were used to fight other aspects of EVD in other locations. At one point MSF had 300 international and 3,000 national staff employed in various EVD treatment units in Guinea, Liberia, and Sierra Leone.

MSF also encountered its limitations during this epidemic. We considered carefully all the above-mentioned options. What ultimately pushed us to close GRC were the obstetrical patients referred from Kenema Government Hospital, where the outbreak was running out of control. The patients we received all had a fever, were bleeding, and had undelivered dead babies still in the uterus. It was a disaster. They had sat in the facility in Kenema for days, cared for by nurses without gloves because none were available.

At that time, the outbreak was progressing so rapidly and out of control that we said, "We have to temporarily close. There is no way MSF can safely [for staff and for patients] guarantee obstetrical care at this time during this outbreak."

What made this decision a little bit easier was that at that time the number of hospital admissions had decreased spectacularly. In the beginning of the outbreak we thought we would have more work and more patients, because the healthcare system was inadequate and falling apart. But the opposite occurred. Unexpectedly we saw fewer patients than before the outbreak. We speculated that the reason for the decrease in patients was that the population was so afraid of contracting EVD in a health facility that they preferred the risk of dying at home.

We closed the obstetric ward in August 2014 at the moment when the outbreak was increasing every day. When, after many discussions and careful considerations, this decision was finally taken, I felt such a mixture of relief and sadness as I never had before. Relief because obstetric care to EVD-positive women was not considered safe. I was worried daily about friends, patients, and coworkers. Sadness because we cut off the lifeline for mothers and babies at the moment when there were no other options in much of the country.

It is the last thing on earth you want to do as a humanitarian, to cut off a lifeline. I knew this decision would mean the death of many mothers and babies. The situation kept me awake at night and haunted me for a long time. For me personally it still is one of the most painful memories of this outbreak.

MSF is committed to improving maternal health in Sierra Leone in the years to come. The plan in the short term was to support health centers with drugs and material and in the medium term, to again provide the emergency obstetrical care as before the outbreak. But the rebuilding of the fragile healthcare system will require much effort and many more part- ners. At this moment there seems to be ample willingness of donors and organizations to assist; hopefully that will continue. I hope, for the people of Sierra Leone, that in five years it will be a better place to be pregnant, to give birth, and to be born. Sometimes miracles happen for those who want to see them. Let's just hope.

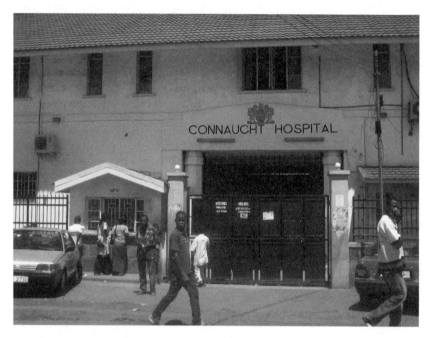

4.1. Connaught Hospital, Freetown, Sierra Leone. Photo courtesy Adam L. Kushner

4

Treating Ebola and Non-Ebola Patients at Connaught Hospital in Freetown, Sierra Leone

THAIM B. KAMARA, MBBS, FWACS

In mid-May 2014 I convened an emergency meeting of the Connaught Hospital Management Committee. News reached Freetown, the capital of Sierra Leone, that Ebola virus disease (EVD) was in the eastern district of Kailahun. This initial meeting led to the selection of a site on the hospital grounds for an eight-bed EVD isolation unit for suspected and confirmed patients. A senior physician was chosen as EVD lead.

A few days later the Sierra Leone Ministry of Health and Sanitation (MOHS) dispatched a delegation headed by the chief nursing officer to assess our preparedness in the event of an EVD outbreak in Freetown. The simple isolation unit was already prepared, and it made a positive impression. EVD was previously unknown locally, and we had no prior experience. The small towns where the outbreak was initially concentrated seemed too far away to be of much concern. We were sadly mistaken.

The following account describes the effect of EVD on the practice of surgery at Connaught Hospital. Connaught is the main adult medical and surgical tertiary referral and teaching hospital in Sierra Leone. Pediatric surgery is also performed there. It has approximately 120 beds.

Before EVD struck in May 2014, the surgical staff comprised six general surgeons, one urologist, and one orthopedic surgeon. These eight specialists were out of only ten fully trained specialist surgeons in the entire country, for a population of over 6 million. Connaught's surgical department included an accident and emergency unit (A&E) and a specialist outpatient clinic (SOP). Trauma and other surgical emergencies were first seen in the A&E and then either discharged home or admitted for specialist care. Patients needing elective surgeries or follow-up after surgery were seen in the SOP.

Before EVD, an average of 30,000 to 36,000 patients were seen annually in the A&E, the SOP, and other specialized clinics. Patients scheduled for surgery were admitted to the surgical wards and then taken to one of two functioning operating rooms on the day of their operation. Initially no dedicated operating room was assigned specifically for EVD-suspected or confirmed patients.

As a government hospital, Connaught is under the supervision of the MOHS. The Management Committee, which I headed, was responsible for the day-to-day functions. Funds and supplies were provided by the MOHS but often arrived late and usually in insufficient quantities. Surgical supplies were basic, with operating room gowns and drapes made of cotton or polyester fabric offering no protection from exposure to blood and fluids. There were limited supplies of examination gloves, plastic aprons, facemasks, and other protective gear. Patients were often evaluated and treated with bare hands. This was the "normal" situation when EVD arrived.

May–July 2014

The first EVD patient at Connaught Hospital was diagnosed in late May 2014. Initially there was minimal impact on the hospital staff. Clinics ran, and surgical operations were performed without any modifications. In July 2014 came news that Dr. Sheik Umar Khan, the young physician in charge of the Lassa Fever Unit, which housed the only PCR laboratory in the country, had tested positive for EVD in Kenema, a city in the eastern province. Like a thunderclap, denial about the existence of EVD evaporated and most healthcare workers and Sierra Leoneans in general started wakening to the truth. If Dr. Khan could contract EVD, then anyone could. A few days later on July 29, 2014, the unthinkable happened, Dr. Sheik Umar Khan died.

Two days before he died the lead physician supervising the isolation unit at Connaught angrily resigned, saying the post should be rotated among surgeons and physicians or given to a junior medical officer. Another physician accepted an offer to collaborate with Kings Sierra Leone Partnership (KSLP), representing the Kings College Global Health Programme, in the running of the unit.

Suddenly, suspected EVD patients poured into Connaught, which had the only isolation unit in the city. The unit quickly expanded from 8 beds to 16 and then to 23. When junior doctors were drafted to review the patients in the unit, they refused to do so, citing a lack of knowledge and skills to work without supervision of a senior clinician. Some senior clinicians who did not want to work in the unit initiated a movement to remove it from the hospital premises. Fear of catching EVD caused confusion, mistrust, and even revolt among healthcare workers, and between them and their patients. The outbreak posed serious administrative problems for management from all sides.

A lack of preparation for the management of EVD patients presenting for treatment left many healthcare workers, and especially junior doctors, feeling vulnerable and helpless. The situation worsened with the persistent news of the deaths of large numbers of healthcare workers in Kailahun and Kenema Districts, the initial epicenters of the outbreak. Social media sites such as WhatsApp and Facebook added a new and potent dimension by posting horrific pictures (many of which were fake) of dead bodies or patients in their death throes or abandoned somewhere to die.

A letter dated July 30, 2014, written by the junior doctors working at Connaught Hospital to me as the hospital care manager, the clinician in charge of the day-to-day administration of the hospital, demanded:

1. Immediate suspension of elective surgeries and outpatient clinics except the A&E
2. Discontinuation of the posting of house officers to the isolation unit
3. Provision of infection prevention and control supplies
4. Provision of blood pressure machines, stethoscopes, thermometers, and sharps containers
5. Training in infection prevention and recognition and management of EVD-suspected patients

An emergency management committee meeting held on July 31 endorsed most of the demands and even went further to impose screening for all patients arriving at the hospital. The resolutions were forwarded to the MOHS for approval and action. From then on, no patients were allowed to see the emergency doctor without having their temperature, pulse, and history of recent travel to the epicenters in Sierra Leone or to Guinea or Liberia taken and documented.

On July 31 a State of Public Health Emergency was declared by the government to stem the spread of the disease. Movement of individuals was restricted, and large social gatherings were banned. Bars and other areas of recreation were forced to close. Furthermore, unlicensed health facilities (known locally as mushroom clinics, as they seemed to sprout up randomly and frequently), pharmacies, and other drug outlets where treatment for both medical and surgical ailments were often provided were also ordered to shut down.

August 2014

By the beginning of August, the MOHS started to deliver sizable quantities of supplies, though personal protective equipment (PPE) for EVD was only available in the isolation unit and not in the operating rooms. Concern was growing on how to protect healthcare workers from contracting EVD while still providing care to the public. We had to ensure that Connaught would not close as so many other private, and even public, facilities had.

From August onward the magnitude of the outbreak became obvious to many as it ravaged almost all regions of the country. The psychological toll on healthcare workers was severe. They witnessed the death of colleagues, including a senior physician infected while working in the isolation unit. Junior doctors and nurses went on strike. Multiple healthcare workers failed to report to work. Patients and healthcare workers were stigmatized and mutual distrust became commonplace. From this time only very ill patients went to the hospital for treatment. Others stayed at home, fearful of getting infected with EVD in the hospital.

After the resignation of the first physician who led the isolation unit and the death of the second, no Sierra Leonean doctor was willing to work there. Most Sierra Leonean doctors did not even want to have the isolation unit on the hospital grounds. Management, however, insisted that it must stay to prevent EVD patients from getting admitted to the regular wards and spreading the disease to other patients and healthcare workers and thereby forcing the closure of the hospital. Finally, KSLP agreed to run the isolation unit.

The symptoms of EVD are in many ways common to those of many routine surgical conditions with fever, abdominal pain, vomiting, and intestinal bleeding. This caused a significant challenge, because any patient presenting with these symptoms had to be kept in the isolation unit even though they might not be EVD-positive. With only 23 beds, empty beds in the unit became a critical factor determining the number of patients allowed to see the emergency doctor on a given day. Therefore, only patients with open wounds and trauma victims were given unfettered access to the emergency doctor.

At the height of the outbreak, the only PCR laboratory to diagnose EVD was in Kenema, over 300 kilometers from Freetown. It took three to five days or even longer to get results. During this time only one ambulance was equipped to transport EVD-suspected patients for testing or treatment. The roads were bad; some patients died along the way. Patients who could not be transferred for testing or care and who could not be determined to be EVD- negative had to wait. Frequently these undiagnosed patients were ill from non-EVD conditions such as a perforated stomach ulcer or appendicitis. Patients suffered and some died.

With no PPE in the operating rooms, the surgeons decided to avoid doing abdominal surgeries until patients tested negative for EVD. Some surgeons advocated for routine testing of all patients. Trust between physicians and patients plummeted. Physicians believed patients were deliberately lying about their symptoms so that they could be seen at the A&E. All patients had to be treated as possibly infected with EVD.

For example, when a 65-year-old man presented at the A&E complaining of an inability to urinate for some days, the examination was in compliance with an informal "no-touch" policy stemming from the physicians' lack of trust in the patients. This patient was sent to the trauma ward and the surgeon-on-call was contacted to evaluate him. Standing some distance away, the surgeon asked, "Did you receive treatment before coming here?" The answer was an affirmative, saying he had received six liters of intravenous fluids in a health center. Asked why he was given intravenous fluids, the patient said he had vomited many times and also had episodes of diarrhea. He did not give a history of exposure to EVD. The surgeon subsequently put on protective gear and passed a urinary catheter. There was no urine in the patient's bladder. The patient was transferred to the isolation unit, where he tested positive for EVD and later died.

Just as some patients presenting to the hospital truly had EVD, others did not and were sick with appendicitis, perforated duodenal ulcers, abscesses, or fractures. The problem, however, was many of the patients did not believe that EVD was real and did not see any reason why they should change their behavior or their practices or even tell the truth to their caregiver.

Other challenges ensued. Quarantines used to halt the spread of EVD trapped patients in their communities. A 9-year-old boy who fell from a tree and broke his forearm needed to wait several days for the quarantine to be lifted before his family could take him to the hospital. When he finally arrived, his arm was gangrenous and had to be amputated.

The rising number of deaths among healthcare workers caused a devastating blow to their colleagues. Morale was low, and families prevailed on loved ones to stop working and stay at home. To improve safety and strengthen the confidence of healthcare workers and reassure the public, the MOHS, in collaboration with international organizations, initiated a series of trainings for all cadres of healthcare workers.

All the surgeons at Connaught attended at least two sessions, the first organized by Public Health England and the other by the International Organization for Migration. The trainings played a positive role in changing the attitudes of healthcare workers to PPE. It is important to note, however, that while the PPE provided protection, inappropriate use contributed to the contamination of several healthcare workers who later became ill and died.

Initially, screening of patients was done in the outpatient department area on the hospital grounds. Instead of protecting healthcare workers this practice actually brought them face to face with EVD-suspected patients. When the isolation unit was full—either because patients' results had not arrived back from Kenema or there was nowhere to take those who tested positive for treatment or there was no ambulance to transport them—then the A&E stopped functioning.

Screening patients in the outpatient department meant keeping large crowds of very sick patients roaming about the interior hospital courtyard in close contact with healthcare workers and visitors. Some vomited, defecated, and died while waiting to see the emergency doctor.

September 2014

A flood of sick patients occurred after the first three-day lockdown enforced by the government in September 2014. The aim was to encourage families and communities to take their sick loved ones out of their homes and bring them to the hospitals. Almost all private hospitals had at this time closed down; those that were still open sent almost all their patients to Connaught. We were thus completely overwhelmed. The government could not allow such a scene at the entrance of its flagship hospital, and it exerted immense pressure on management to move the isolation unit somewhere from within the hospital compound. This made it possible for patients to freely access the physicians.

There was nowhere else to move the isolation unit. In consultation with KSLP and with approval from the MOHS, management decided to construct two screening tents in front of the main hospital gate. Patients could now wait and get screened in the tents before they were seen by the emergency doctor. This innovation did not cut down on the time spent waiting to see the doctor but did improve privacy and safety.

While the isolation unit had almost everything it needed to handle EVD-suspected or confirmed cases, the rest of the hospital did not. There was a need for large quantities of rubber boots, scrubs, and other supplies for infection prevention and control. In September 2014, Surgeons Over-Seas, a US-based surgical capacity–building organization which had collaborated with Connaught and the MOHS since 2008, made a donation of US$5,000. The money was used to purchase boots, scrubs, hand sanitizers, and other locally available infection prevention and control items. That gesture went a long way to alleviate the problem of inadequate supplies for surgeons at that time.

Testing for EVD in patients presenting with surgical conditions became controversial and caused significant disagreements between surgeons on the one hand and isolation unit workers and phlebotomists on the other. Management was forced to intervene in some of these disputes. It was initially agreed that only patients presenting with symptoms similar to EVD needed to be tested. Soon, however, especially as doctors and nurses started dying from the disease, the surgeons demanded that EVD tests be done on all patients. This demand for routine testing for all patients was not helpful. Without symptoms consistent with EVD, what would one be testing for? What about the time it took to get back a result, three to five days or more? What about false positives or false negatives? Waiting for these tests caused unnecessary delays in surgery for emergency conditions, and delays were known to cause worse outcomes in many cases.

The disagreements were transiently settled by the guidelines developed by Drs. Sherry Wren and Adam Kushner. (For more detail see Chapter 1.) However, they were not uniformly endorsed, because they did not originate from the World Health Organization. Also, the isolation unit workers were developing their own guidelines, but since there was no surgeon among them little regarding surgical care was included.

October–November 2014

In October, one of the house officers with a fever was isolated. He spent a week in the unit before his negative result came back. Initially the first blood specimen was lost and a new one had to be sent, but luckily additional testing facilities were set up and turnaround time was reduced. He was finally released from the isolation unit.

Fear still influenced care. For example, a young woman was admitted to the ward with breast cancer and a need for surgery. She was kept on the ward for over 21 days, the length of time, most experts agree, within which an exposure to EVD will manifest. Even after this time, with no signs of infection and no fever, the surgeon still insisted on an EVD test. This occurred despite a rapidly growing tumor, which was at the point of breaking through her skin.

The vulnerability of the operating room staff to EVD—in view of the lack of adequate PPE and drapes—was brought to the notice of the chief medical officer at the MOHS. Through his efforts a quantity of cooling vests, freezers, and other accessories were donated to all the hospitals in the country, including Connaught. The cooling vests were intended for use by staff of the isolation unit and operating rooms, though, from personal experience, their use in the operation room was not a priority. The PPE, which was used in the isolation units and which was later supplied to the operating rooms, was very hot. Without some form of cooling, it was uncomfortable and hard to tolerate for longer than one hour without getting exhausted or dehydrated. The cooling vests were loaded with nine ice packs, six in the front and three behind.

While the PPE was suitable for use in isolation units, in the operating room, the combination of PPE and cooling vest was fraught with challenges. The PPE was not sterile; traditional scrubbing was impossible while in PPE; and since our operating rooms were not air-conditioned and the weather was hot, sweating was a problem. Also, the PPE recommended by

Wren and Kushner, AAMI level 4, was not available in our hospital and too expensive to procure.

December 2014

By December 2014 four doctors, among them one physician, two surgeons, and one medical officer, had died at Connaught. Fifteen nurses, porters, and cleaners also died. The two surgeons died less than four weeks apart. No one knew for certain how or where they got infected. It is important to highlight, however, the difficulty of putting up an effective counterattack against EVD and to caution those who hastily advocate for surgery in patients who test positive for the disease. One of the surgeons had symptoms consistent with EVD but initially tested negative. When he did not improve, a second test was ordered two days later. That test was positive. He ultimately was transferred to the United States for care but died shortly after arrival in Nebraska. (For more details see Chapter 2.)

The second surgeon's symptoms were not initially consistent with EVD, as he presented with visual problems and ophthalmoplegia (paralysis or weakness of the eye muscles) and received treatment for a prior medical condition he was known to have. The death of these two surgeons, both colleagues and friends of mine, the equivalent of 20% of Sierra Leone's surgeons, was a devastating blow both personally and to the overall health system.

The danger of spreading EVD while caring for colleagues is real and must be kept in mind. The loss of these two surgeons, one who was just 44 years old, was disastrous and will be hard to replace. Fortunately, none of the doctors and other caregivers who treated these two surgeons was infected, but that was a serious concern, since they were initially admitted to a regular ward and to the intensive care unit.

These deaths also contributed greatly to the precautionary attitudes adopted by their remaining colleagues. The number of surgeries performed in December 2014 tumbled to just 3% of preoutbreak levels, and admissions to the surgical wards fell by an average of 35%.

February 2015

Eventually protocols were finalized, and from February 2015 all surgical procedures at Connaught were performed with all operating room staff dressed in full PPE, either with or without cooling vests.

The government and its international partners must be commended for mobilizing large amounts of local and international resources and for setting up several isolation and treatment centers, laboratories for testing, and cutting the turnaround time of test results from several days to 24 hours. Fleets of ambulances and other vehicles dedicated to burying the dead were brought in by air and sea. All these interventions contributed to the reduction in the number of new cases and deaths.

May 2015

In May 2015, with a decrease in the countrywide numbers of EVD-positive patients, the pressure on Connaught eased, though patient visits to the A&E began to increase to preoutbreak levels. In spite of these developments and with the resumption of the more normal care, the operating room restrictions on elective surgeries were not removed. Preparations were needed for the large numbers of elective surgical patients waiting for treatment, since elective surgical operations were suspended in July 2014.

Prevention, they say, is better than cure. Perhaps if the entire Kissidougou area in Kailahun District, where the outbreak began, was quickly quarantined at the start, the country would have been spared much of the horror. The Nigerians taught all the affected countries a lesson they should not soon forget, namely, aggressive contact tracing by surveillance teams. Finally, by the time this outbreak is declared over, there must be universally acceptable guidelines for surgical practice during EVD outbreaks. In the future such guidelines will help surgeons, along with the outcome of the current EVD vaccine trial in the region, to continue providing surgical care in a safe and sound manner, even during outbreaks.

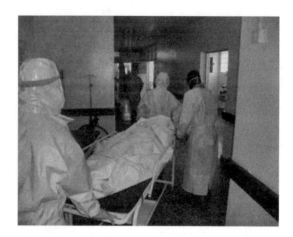

5.1. A maternal death from Ebola in the out-
patient operation room at Princess Christian
Maternity Hospital, Freetown, Sierra Leone.
Photo courtesy Michael Koroma

5

Anesthesia and Ebola

A Loss of Touch

EVA HANCILES, MD, FWACS, MARK J. HARRIS, MD, MPH, AND
MICHAEL KOROMA, MD, FWACS

Ebola strikes at the very heart of the humanistic interaction—touch. In the world of anesthesia the ability to touch patients not only fulfills this human prerogative but also provides us with invaluable information. Is our patient too hot or too cold? How is his pulse? Is she breathing deeply enough?

In the wealthy operating suites of the United States and Western Europe this "hands-on" medicine is replaced by sophisticated (and greatly beneficial) monitoring systems. The nations struck by Ebola virus disease (EVD) had few of these advanced monitors. Tragically, EVD removed touch, the most common, simple, vital mode of assessment and reassurance.

As discussed elsewhere, providing surgical care for a patient with suspected EVD puts healthcare workers at risk. Such care should only be done when the benefits significantly outweigh the risks. The patient must also have a meaningful chance of survival.

At the height of the EVD outbreak in Sierra Leone, the Princess Christian Maternity Hospital (PCMH) in Freetown, the main government tertiary and referral center for maternal care in the country, was the only facility offering uninterrupted obstetric services. Before the epidemic, cases that could not be managed in other facilities were referred to PCMH. Ordinarily, 90% of these referral cases required surgery for problems such as prolonged and obstructed labor, intrauterine fetal death, uterine rupture, or septic shock. To complicate matters, most of these conditions require surgery even if EVD is suspected.

During the EVD outbreak, patients were fearful that healthcare workers might be infected, or even deliberately spreading the disease. Consequently, many patients only came to a hospital when severely ill, often too late for successful intervention. Even if patients presented earlier, they were often uncooperative with staff. This hindered the ability of anesthetists to carry out adequate preoperative assessments, limited necessary preparations, and increased the chances of operative complications. Such unwarranted suspicion and paranoia undermined the fundamental aspects of every healthcare interaction. Without the trust of a patient, a healthcare worker is severely hindered in undertaking their duties. In addition, fear of contracting EVD from patients often hampered appropriate care by the physicians and nurses.

EVD isolation and treatment units did not routinely have anesthesia or surgical staff present. Therefore, EVD-suspected patients who needed surgery suffered delays in their preoperative workup and management. This was as basic (but important) as pain control and as vital as the timely cleaning of a wound to prevent an amputation.

The incubation period for EVD is between 2 and 21 days of infection. During this period a patient with EVD is asymptomatic but still able to transmit the virus through blood or other body fluids. Therefore, it is important for surgical staff to know the test status of their patients. Unfortunately the tests available in Sierra Leone during the outbreak could take from two to five days to come back. Urgent surgical cases were often sent to the operating room without definitive test results, and the staff would operate under the assumption that the patient was EVD-positive.

Procedures commonly performed by anesthesia staff include intubation, the placing of a breathing tube in the airway. These procedures are in the mouth and throat of a patient and can generate aerosolized saliva particles, which can expose the operating room staff to EVD. Disturbing data by Missair et al. implied that exposure to these aerosolized particles resulted in a greater degree of infection compared to infection from other types of transmission. The American Society of Anesthesiologists Ebola Workgroup explicitly recommended enhanced personal protective equipment (PPE) to prevent exposure to EVD via aerosolized particles during such procedures and throughout surgery. The recommended equipment included sophisticated respirators with full facemask, disposable hoods that extend to the shoulders, triple gloves, impermeable and washable shoes, impermeable shoe covers, and duct tape over seams.

During the EVD outbreak sophisticated respirators were never available in Sierra Leone; most of the other equipment was, albeit intermittently. When PPE was unavailable, elective cases were postponed until EVD tests on the patients proved negative. Many patients refused to be tested, fearing the stigma of a positive diagnosis. The resulting delay (or cancellation) of surgery potentially worsened their condition.

Debates as to the type of anesthesia to be used ensued. It was suggested that with the possible exposure to contaminated droplets and aerosols, and the complexity of sterilization of intricate machinery, intubation and ventilation should always be avoided in favor of regional "nerve-blocking" anesthetic techniques. Regional anesthetic techniques are not without risks and include exposure to needles, with studies showing that needle stick injuries with EVD can result in death.

With transmission of the virus higher during the fever stage, healthcare workers were advised to treat all patients with a fever and any signs or symptoms of EVD as if they were infected. Staff exposed to infected fluids such as sputum, vomitus, or blood had the exposed area washed with chlorine solution and were quarantined and observed for 21 days before returning to work. Healthcare workers who did not observe strict universal precautions during procedures usually became infected with the virus; many died.

In the summer of 2014, with many healthcare workers in Sierra Leone dying from EVD, most of the junior doctors stopped working and isolated themselves. Consequently, almost every case requiring obstetric surgery in the country was referred to the PCMH and increased the demands on the remaining staff.

In the setting of an EVD outbreak, the US Centers for Disease Control and Prevention (CDC) recommended using disposable equipment whenever possible. Unfortunately, in most developing countries such as Sierra Leone, such throwaway equipment was not available. Therefore at PCMH, all equipment was disinfected using chlorine solution. Gear that was truly disposable was burned, as per protocol. Initially, supplies of proper PPE, training, and knowledge were inadequate to guide anesthesia decisions during this difficult time.

Like everyone else in the country caring for sick patients, we tried to do the best we could with the supplies at hand. As the epidemic progressed and ultimately came under control, safety for healthcare workers and care for patients improved. (For more on developments at PCMH, see Chapter 7.) We can only hope that the lessons of this outbreak will be learned and that the health system can be strengthened to avoid future epidemics.

ADDITIONAL READING

American Society of Anesthesiologists Ebola information. *http://www.asahq.org /resources/clinical-information/ebola-information* (accessed July 12, 2015).

Carrol MW, Matthews DA, Hiscox JA, et al. Temporal and spatial analysis of the 2014-2015 Ebola virus outbreak in West Africa. *Nature*. June 17, 2015.

Günther S, Feldmann H, Geisbert TW, et al. Management of accidental exposure to Ebola virus in the biosafety level 4 laboratory, Hamburg, Germany. *J Infect Dis* 2011;204 Suppl 3:S785-90.

Missair A, Marino MJ, Vu CN, et al. Anesthetic implications of Ebola patient management: a review of the literature and policies. *Anesthesia & Analgesia*, Dec. 30, 2014.

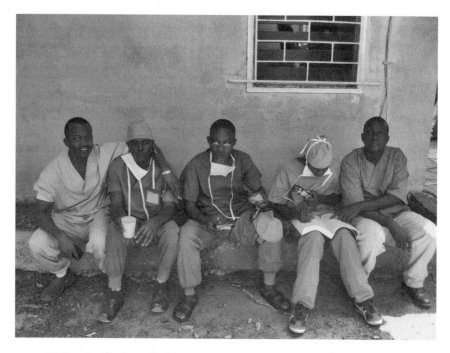

6.1. Surgical trainees in Sierra Leone. Photo courtesy Håkon A. Bolkan

6

How Ebola Affected a Clinical Officer Training Program in Sierra Leone and the Decline of Surgical Care

HÅKON A. BOLKAN, MD

In 2012, community health officer Samuel Batty applied for surgical training with CapaCare, a Norwegian nongovernmental organization working in Sierra Leone. In his application, he wrote:

> I am interested in this course for the following reasons: A lot of disasters and crises are facing our rural populations in Sierra Leone. Due to limited surgical and obstetric skills among health providers and poor functioning of health facilities, obstetric and surgical emergencies cost many lives and disabilities. Only a handful of consultant surgeons and obstetricians are available in Sierra Leone to serve a population of more than six million and nearly all of them are based in the capital city, Freetown. The rural and hard to reach areas are left abandoned. It is in this vein I have deemed it necessary to strive hard to tap any possible opportunity to be trained in obstetric and surgical emergencies to help reduce child and maternal mortality in our country.

In November 2014 he assisted a pregnant woman with a fever. She had responded to antimalarial medications and it was assumed she had malaria. After a busy 24-hour shift he reexamined her without full personal protective equipment (PPE). It was a fatal mistake. One week later he, too, developed a fever and on December 2 died of confirmed Ebola virus disease (EVD). He was only a few weeks away from completing the CapaCare Surgical Training Program (STP).

Surgical care is difficult to obtain in Sierra Leone, and few people receive the operations they need. In the United States approximately 10,000 operations are performed each year for every 100,000 people; however, in Sierra

Leone only 400 cases are done per 100,000. In 2012 fewer than 25,000 major operations were performed. To address this problem, the STP was created to increase the number of healthcare workers in rural areas with surgical skills. Initiated in 2011, the plan was by 2019 to train 60 physicians and community health officers to work in the country's district hospitals. After finishing the program, graduates would be able to handle most common surgical and obstetrical emergencies that without treatment would lead to death or disability.

STP students first trained for six to nine months at the Masanga Hospital in Tonkolili District. They then did six-month rotations at partner hospitals throughout the country. During the initial two years of the program, each student participated in 650 to 1,000 major operations. In 2013 STP students participated in a total of 7,000 major operations, nearly 30% of all procedures in Sierra Leone. By May 2015, five students had graduated with another 37 in training.

With students spread throughout Sierra Leone, the EVD outbreak had major implications for the STP. Beginning in April 2014, Masanga Hospital prepared for the possibility of infected patients. PPE was ordered, triage and isolation areas were constructed, and guidelines were developed.

Early in the outbreak, a student assigned in Kenema, in the eastern region of Sierra Leone where EVD was first identified, wrote:

> June 12: With the trend of the Ebola outbreak, patients are not coming to the hospital so there is not much surgical activity. Very little PPE is found on the wards. We touch unknowingly confirmed cases and it happens almost everyday. I'm kindly requesting for a re-posting to another hospital. I'm worried for my safety, as no one knows who is infected or not. Secondary, no one knows when the epidemic will stop. By then, the skills I have acquired might disappear, so please sir, consider my re-posting. Above all I'm really worried about my safety as I'm almost every day feverish.

The student was reassigned to another hospital in a district without reported EVD cases.

By late July the PPE had still not arrived at Masanga Hospital. Without protective gear, with an increase in EVD cases, and with patients not always providing full EVD contact histories and passing through the triage, the hospital was forced to close. We had to acknowledge that we were not able to safely provide for the staff, and we did not have the resources to run an EVD isolation or treatment center. All the students in the first part of their training were offered temporary paid leave. At the same time we contacted all the students at our partner hospitals, shared our EVD protocols, requested that they observe strict infection prevention control, and only take part in clinical activity of surgical and obstetrical patients if proper triage and protection was available.

In August things got worse. One student in Freetown wrote:

August 9: I am personally worried about our training as a candidate in the Surgical Training Program simply because of the ongoing spread of the Ebola virus. I have lost 3 of my uncles to Ebola. As I speak now, there are over five of my family members admitted at the treatment center in Kailahun. It's really not an easy moment for me. Hearing about mortality due to Ebola every day really pulls me down which is affecting the efficiency of my work as a student. Even the caseload now has reduced rapidly because patients are scared of coming to the hospital saying we the health workers are the carriers of the virus. I have not come in contact with any Ebola case and I do not want to.

Even though international organizations are contributing greatly to combat the spread, still there are multiple challenges. You can imagine the hospital where I'm working presently, not up to 20% of the staff have had any training in infection control. There are also limited medical consumables, poor isolation systems, and inadequate infrastructure for health staff. These and many more are the main reason for the rapid spread of the virus amongst health care givers. Even today we had a senior physician positive, can you imagine?

With these challenges and the risk involved in executing my duty, my family is crying every day and asks me to stop visiting the hospital premises, as I mean a lot to them. Presently "After the Lord, you are our hope," says my father. "Your living is more paramount." But my question is, "Who is to do the work now father?"

I am therefore asking on all of you to please join hands together to help fight this deadly disease in our nation, as you have been supporting hard to see the success of the Surgical Training Program [sic]. Now it's an urgent need. Even our training is shaky. Thank you all for patiently going through this message."

A few days later another student, also in Freetown, wrote:

August 12: I write to keep you informed about my situation in the hospital I have been assigned. There is a good relationship between the entire staff and me and more especially with Dr. Martin Salia [Dr. Salia later contracted Ebola and was transported to the Nebraska Biocontainment Unit, where he died. For more details, see Chapter 2], who is directly supervising my work. In spite of the Ebola crisis and a very worrying situation, I have still continued to work. Attendance rate for surgical cases has drastically dropped in the health care facilities across the entire country.

At the moment, no modality has been put in place to deal appropriately with any suspected case at the point of entry to the hospital. I feel that the entire staff is at risk of this illness, since we now have a handful of cases in the city. My own risk is further compounded by the use of public transport, which is very much congested, and further more, one has to scramble before getting into the vehicle. I have tried to get a place very close to the hospital to no avail. I will keep you informed with any new update.

Later in the month, a message arrived concerning Joseph Ngegba, an STP student based in Makeni:

August 20: Hello Dr. I'm very sorry to inform you that Joseph is admitted in a hospital now for the past four days with high fever, abdominal pain, vomiting, anorexia, body weakness and a sore throat. He was positive for malaria and typhoid and has been on treatment for the past days, but he is still having fever. So I advised the management to collect a blood sample and send it to Kenema to rule out Ebola. Dr. I'm really confused and you really need to pray for us.

August 21, morning: Joseph is dying. He is not improving. We want to take him to Kenema, but there is no vehicle available.

August 21, afternoon: It is with a heartfelt cry to inform you that we have lost our colleague Joseph.

The blood sample from Joseph confirmed EVD. During his hospitalization, his father visited him. We later learned that both Joseph's wife and father contracted EVD and died; fortunately, his brother and sister survived. Joseph was only 29 years old. His 1-year-old son became one of the many EVD orphans and was now cared for by his extended family.

With Joseph's death, it became clear that the safeguards against EVD in partner hospitals were unsatisfactory. We stopped all clinical training. This was a difficult decision, given the signals it would send to other healthcare workers and the need for manpower. The STP students, with their on-the-job training, were key personnel in these facilities and contributed substantially to the daily clinical work. Despite the need, the goal of the STP program was to build capacity in surgery and obstetrics, and this could no longer be accomplished. What helped make the decision easier was the sharp decrease in the number of operations performed by STP students.

As the number of cases fell, CapaCare, with approval of the Sierra Leone Ministry of Health and Sanitation, began a surveillance initiative to monitor effects of the outbreak on surgical services. Sixty-one government and private facilities that offered major surgery, defined as a surgical procedure under anesthesia and performed within an operating room, were surveyed. The community health officers temporarily taken out of the STP were trained in data collection and visited the facilities. Weekly data from operating room logbooks were available from 40 facilities. Baseline was defined as the weeks prior to the first reported EVD case on May 26, 2014.

The survey documented a total of 15,848 major procedures performed in 2014. Initially the facilities performed on average 9.8 procedures per week. In the final 11 weeks of 2014, institutions averaged only 4 procedures per week—a 60% decrease from baseline. For much of early 2015, the number of surgical procedures remained low, and it was not until the spring that hospitals resumed operative procedures.

In May 2015 Masanga Hospital reopened. Seven new STP students started with theoretical training and a skills lab. At the same time, Emmanuel Tommy, the first community health officer to complete the three-year training, wrote about his experience with EVD. His story began in June 2014 as he waited to be posted to a governmental hospital.

> It started at the early phase of the outbreak of the Ebola disease, when I was contacted by Serabu Hospital to cover the surgical department for emergency surgical conditions for the first three weeks of July 2014. Surgeons from abroad used to come to the hospital on regular rotations to take care of the surgical patients. Because of the Ebola outbreak, they stopped coming and the hospital was left without anyone to take care of the surgical patients.
>
> This was my first challenge after completing my internship. I had to take this offer to test myself. In the hospital I organized the day to day running of the surgical activities. It was challenging for me. I had to make critical surgical decisions, but was ready to take responsibility of the outcome. I had to work

very hard, often 24-hours round the clock to achieve my objectives. Due to the good working relationship with my team and the entire staff I got the support I needed. As it was uncertain when the international surgeons could return, the hospital management asked me to stay.

I had to extend my surgical activities by undertaking elective surgical conditions within capability. I had a small surgical outpatient consultation room that ran daily from 1 p.m. to 4 p.m., Mondays to Fridays. Besides that I performed acute operations when needed. On Saturdays and Sundays we only did emergencies. As I was the only skilled surgical provider in the hospital, I was always on call to take care of the emergencies. I did ward rounds every morning to review my surgical patients. It continued like this until November when the highest incidence and mortality of Ebola was recorded. Several of my fellow health workers all over the country had at that time contracted the disease and died. This was the climax of the whole situation.

Our chiefdom, Bumpe, became at one time an Ebola hot spot. Over 30 people contracted the disease and many died in a village about 25 km from our hospital. There were also other surrounding catchment areas with Ebola cases. We were all scared of this disease visiting our hospital. During this period we decided to close the surgical department. However, we had to ask ourselves: "Are we able to watch our pregnant women die of obstructed labor or a ruptured uterus? Are we able to watch a young healthy teenage boy die of typhoid bowel perforation or a young man in his early thirties die of obstructed or strangulated hernia because we were scared of Ebola?" We said, "NO!!!!"

Then let's keep on the fight. We decided to limit our number of operations and concentrate on attending to only emergencies, mostly obstetrics. We were able to put in place standard protocols in the hospital; use of PPE, a triage system for the identification of suspected Ebola cases, and an Ebola identification strategy in the wards. The operation room was well equipped with PPE. We had to accept some risks to be able to help our people in need of these services. We stayed in this war front till now. In January another colleague from the STP program replaced me for 2 weeks, and I could get some rest.

Serabu became the only functional hospital with surgical capability in this part of the district. Surgical cases were referred from the neighboring districts, Bonthe and Moyamba and even from Bo town, the second largest city in Sierra Leone.

As of May 2015, I carried out 271 operations during the Ebola outbreak. About

80% of them were emergencies. The majority of the emergencies were related to obstetric care. Obstetric hemorrhage, placenta previa, abrution, ruptured uterus, cervical tear, postpartum hysterectomy, retained placenta, incomplete abortions, and ruptured ectopic pregnancies were most common. I also attended many with obstructed labor and mal-presentations that could be solved without performing surgery. The most common general surgical conditions were obstructed or strangulated hernias, typhoid bowel perforations, traumatic bowel perforations, gastric perforation, intestinal obstruction, acute urinary retention, and major lacerations. I performed hernia repairs, bowel resections and anastomosis, thoracic drainage, drained abscesses, etc. The elective cases were mainly hernia repairs, myomectomies, ovarian cystectomies, and a range of minor surgical interventions.

To my knowledge, the outcomes so far were good. I did not record a death of a patient as a result of failure of responsibility on my part, due to my decision-making, or the surgical intervention. I must admit, it was a hard time and a lot of work. But this ten months spell in the hospital also earned me a great deal of experience in emergency surgery and obstetrics. It became clear to me that I must improve my skills and competence level every day, so I can be more confident and take on further responsibilities. It was rewarding to use my skills to serve my people and this has also given me more ambition for further academic pursuance.

The near future for everybody involved with surgical care in Sierra Leone will be a challenge. Patients will be reluctant to go to hospitals out of fear of EVD, and possibly this will continue for a long time after the outbreak is contained. Any responsible employer of a surgical unit must put in place measures to ensure the safety of patients and staff. Screening and reliable testing of patients for EVD and supply of adequate PPE will remain important. All the extra measurements will most likely add costs to healthcare. This will make surgery unaffordable for a larger proportion of the population, and the rural poor will again be the most affected. Many psychological barriers, both among patients and healthcare workers need to be addressed to restore confidence in surgical services.

Training the next generation of surgical providers in Sierra Leone will also be a challenge, as case volume is needed to learn surgery. We hope the international community recognizes the breakdown of the healthcare systems in the EVD-affected West African countries. Larger involvement from many actors is needed to strengthen the system. We at CapaCare will continue in the words of our late student, Samuel Batty: "We will strive hard to tap any possible opportunity to offer high quality training in obstetrics and surgery to reduce child and maternal mortality in Sierra Leone."

ADDITIONAL READING

Bolkan HA, Bash-Taqi DA, Samai M, Gerdin M, von Schreeb J. Ebola and indirect effects on health service function in Sierra Leone. *PLoS Curr.* 2014 Dec 19;6.

Bolkan HA, von Schreeb J, Samai MM, Bash-Taqi DA, Kamara TB, Salvesen Ø, Ystgaard B, Wibe A. Met and unmet needs for surgery in Sierra Leone: a comprehensive, retrospective, countrywide survey from all health care facilities performing operations in 2012. *Surgery.* 2015 Jun;157(6):992-1001.

III TECHNICAL CONSIDERATIONS AND A WAY FORWARD

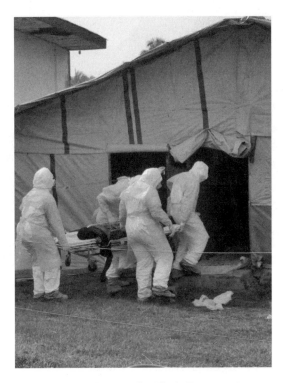

Admitting a patient to the Ebola Treatment Unit, Greenville, Liberia. Photo courtesy Joseph Forrester

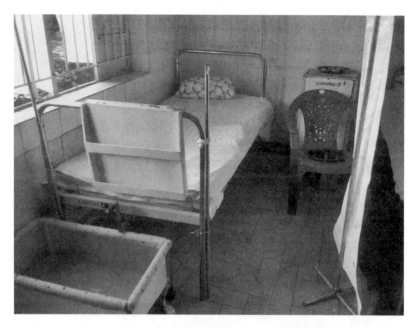

7.1. Ebola isolation room at Princess Christian Maternity Hospital, Freetown, Sierra Leone. Photo courtesy Andrew M. R. Hall

7

Maternity Care during the

West African Ebola Outbreak

ANDREW M. R. HALL, DIPHE, ANDREW J. MICHAELS, MD, MPH,
FACS, KATHRYN P. BARRON, NP, MARTA LADO, MD, DTMH

The Kings College Sierra Leone Partnership (KSLP) pioneered a model of creating and supporting quick-to-build, temporary Ebola virus disease (EVD) isolation facilities at multiple public health units (small primary care facilities) and hospitals in Sierra Leone. By November 2014 they supported nearly 90 beds in the Western Area of Freetown. After four months of working with EVD-suspected and positive patients, Partners In Health (PIH), a US-based nongovernmental organization, asked for assistance to build an isolation unit for EVD-suspected and positive mothers at the Princess Christian Maternity Hospital (PCMH) in Freetown.

For months, PCMH staff dealt with suspected EVD patients on their own with some success. One major accomplishment was the successful delivery of a child born from an EVD-positive mother. The child survived. It was a situation never before seen, and it inspired hope.

Although the number of mothers referred to PCMH to deliver did not significantly drop during the outbreak, the level of care was impacted by many factors. Initially the staff lacked confidence and experience with EVD. PCMH lacked basic quantities of personal protective equipment (PPE) and a supply chain to back up day-to-day functions. With a lack of support also came a lack of organization, leading some nurses to work long hours inside the isolation facility and increase their risk of making a mistake due to exhaustion.

In August 2014 training was provided to the PCMH maternity staff in the use of PPE and how to manage suspected patients. In November 2014, building upon this limited experience, we created a dedicated, temporary EVD isolation unit, constructed with timber and tarpaulins.

How were conditions improved in this difficult setting? The answer was to establish a supportive environment with high-level maternity care delivered by experienced nurses and midwives and to provide the systems for them to perform safely. The majority of admissions to the maternity unit were women in labor who met EVD case definition with common symptoms: fever, abdominal pain, diarrhea, and vomiting. Many colleagues outside of PCMH expressed grave concern about working with EVD-positive pregnant women. They stated that it was the most dangerous thing a clinician could do. With so much blood and bodily fluid, it was thought to be almost impossible not to have a PPE breach while working or during the doffing procedure. Before the establishment of the PCMH isolation unit, numerous healthcare workers at other facilities had died while delivering children from EVD-positive mothers.

Before the isolation unit was established and guidelines and protocols put in place, many staff were fearful and suspicious of suspected patients. The stigma of coming from a high-risk area, or even from an area unknown to the staff, frequently resulted in the refusal to provide care. Often patients were abandoned on the floor or on benches in full view of petrified passersby.

During the first week of December 2014, we were given a building on the hospital grounds, made structural adaptations and trained the national staff. The first priority was to establish a safe place to work and a formal system to care for patients. The building, a converted radiology department, had been empty for many months. We used temporary fencing to isolate the structure from the rest of the hospital. We created separate contained drainage for wastewater and a sealed waste removal trolley to remove waste for incineration. Everything apart from the waste incinerator was contained within the isolation unit.

Using one-way doors and protocols, a one-way-only flow was created. Hand washing stations were set up in each area along with extra gloves and aprons to allow staff to decontaminate and change their gloves and aprons between patients.

We created individual patient bays consisting of: a bed, a commode, and a bedside cabinet/table. This helped to stop patients from interacting too closely with each other and reduced the risk of spreading infection through the use of shared facilities. The unit was further divided into three distinct areas: a low-risk area of six beds; a high-risk area of three beds; and two separate delivery rooms entirely self-contained—effectively isolation rooms within an isolation facility. Once this was completed, we began receiving patients.

All areas needed continuous mentorship, both clinical and nonclinical, but we always worked together. We learned that working for KSLP meant, "No one is too senior to mop floors, wash patients, or move corpses." We led by example.

Within weeks of opening we were able to safely isolate and provide high-level care to maternity patients at all stages of their pregnancy. We regularly delivered children from suspected and confirmed EVD-positive mothers while wearing full PPE in 30+ degrees centigrade (86+ degrees Fahrenheit) with 100% humidity.

Providing basic care in these conditions was difficult. We wore category III suits, double gloved, put on N95 facemasks, face shields, and impermeable aprons. All this was over rubber boots and scrubs. It ensured that we lost liters of body fluids and electrolytes every hour. Therefore, it was essential to take in liters of oral rehydration solutions after exiting the isolation area to avoid cramps, headaches, and heat stroke. Staff often finished the day in a condition nearly requiring hospitalization. To help combat the heat, we trialed the use of cooling vests, but the weight often made them too uncomfortable to wear. Also, they would quickly lose their effect and become just another layer to keep in heat. We installed air conditioning but it was ineffective with the fabric walls and the unreliable power supply.

On admission to the isolation unit, patients would be reassured as best as possible. Patients often wrongly assumed that because international staff were working there, that it signified an international healthcare system. It was only later that they realized the inequality they faced. They would receive an initial level of case management to treat symptoms and an assessment of their pregnancy, including vaginal exams. With poor light and inappropriate beds, staff would have to take huge risks to provide care. If patients arrived in labor they would be taken inside to one of two dedicated delivery rooms. These provided an added physical barrier to protect the patients and others from potentially infective pathogens and body fluids.

Nevertheless, often four or five patients would be in labor at the same time. They would remain in the beds separated from each other by impermeable plastic curtains; all we could do was hope that they did not cross-infect each other, or us, and that the attempts to create self-contained patient bays would work.

Due to the high number of EVD tests needed and the distance to the lab, at times the result of a patient's test would not arrive for over a week. Effectively this turned our facility from an EVD isolation unit to an EVD treatment unit. It was clear from the outset that turnaround times on patients' tests were causing needless deaths. Fortunately, with the subsequent arrival of a Dutch mobile lab, turnaround times decreased from days and weeks to just a few hours. This undoubtedly saved dozens of lives every week; however, discharging EVD-negative patients to be cared for in the normal hospital had its own challenges. Often these patients remained with the stigma. The regular ward nurses feared that if they cared for these patients they, too, would become infected.

Surgical procedures such as cesarean sections were impossible to carry out. The hospital would not perform surgery on a suspected EVD patient. In the isolation facility, surgery would have been the most dangerous thing to do for both patients and staff, and it was therefore never attempted.

As the isolation unit became more established, PIH began bringing in expat staff with specific knowledge, including midwives and specialist obstetricians. Far from just doing what they could, the local staff began to fight hard for their patients and provided an extremely high level of care. Side by side, the local and international staff would don our PPE and spend upward of three hours at a time inside the unit providing care to pregnant and laboring women. All the time working together and ensuring that one another worked safely. No one went in alone, and staff always buddied up before donning PPE. It was essential to prepare before entering the high-risk area, as one could not simply go back if you forgot something.

Staff would don PPE and check each other before entering. They would take all medications, equipment, and supplies they needed with them when they entered. As many medications as possible were drawn up outside of the high-risk areas to reduce the potential for sharps and needle stick injuries. Nevertheless, this was not always possible due to the often-urgent needs of patients in labor. We liked to state that there was no reason to rush and,

"There's no such thing as an emergency in a Red Zone." In a maternity ward this is not exactly true; however, extra care must be taken, and we had to force ourselves to slow down and be fully prepared. We realized that we could not look after our patients if we, too, became infected.

Interaction with patients and relatives was very important. In many cases attempting to reassure both patients and their relatives that we were doing all we could to save their loved ones was an unachievable goal. Once patients entered the unit they were often too weak to move to the visiting area to be seen again alive. Some patients would enter alive and conversing with their relatives only to die without their family seeing them again. In addition, all deaths in the Western Area had to be interred by burial teams to ensure a safe burial. This process rarely allowed for the family to view the corpse. The looks on the faces of relatives when we explained to them that their loved one died, despite being told that this was the best place for them to be, was difficult.

At the beginning, no effective triage protocol existed for pregnant women and certainly not for those who arrived in active labor. Often it was difficult to even determine if a patient was in labor or was miscarrying, as accurate dates of conception and the term of pregnancy were frequently unknown. We were told that EVD increased the risk of both miscarriage and premature birth, but how could we tell? Unfortunately, we still know so little about EVD and pregnancy.

Despite the constraints and the difficulties, many lives were saved at PCMH. Over 80 successful deliveries occurred in the facility in less than three months. Much of the credit for the survival of these pregnant mothers and children lies with the local staff who stepped up when others stepped back. They refused to believe that caring for EVD-positive pregnant women was a fight that could not be won. The staff at PCMH, like most local healthcare workers across the country, never anticipated the risk of EVD, the possibility of becoming infected, of dying. Most of the staff did not abandon their posts or their patients. For this they will forever have our undying respect.

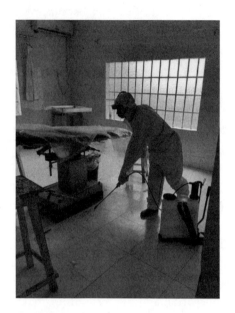

8.1. Cleaning an operating room between cases during Ebola outbreak, Koidu Government Hospital, Kono, Sierra Leone. Photo courtesy Andrew J. Michaels

8

Surgery during a Time of Ebola

ANDREW J. MICHAELS, MD, MPH, FACS, RONALD C. MARSH, MD,
MIPH, MOHAMED G. SHEKU, MD, SONGOR S. J. KOEDOYOMA, MD,
ANDREW M. R. HALL, DIPHE, AND KATHRYN P. BARRON, NP

Drs. Ronald Marsh, Mohamed Sheku, and Songor Koedoyoma grew up in Sierra Leone. They went to medical school in Freetown and trained in a series of government and private hospitals across the country. Typically in the United States it requires five years after medical school to train a general surgeon, but there are no surgical residencies in Sierra Leone. In Sierra Leone, as in much of the developing world, surgeons are not the only people who do surgical operations. Physicians, clinical officers, nurses, and variously trained paramedical personnel learn and develop surgical expertise that is often inconceivable to a specialist from a high-income country.

Before Ebola virus disease (EVD) arrived in Sierra Leone, Drs. Marsh, Sheku, and Koedoyoma performed hundreds of operations a year at the Koidu Government Hospital (KGH) in the small western town of Kono. They were very good at what they did. Remarkably, during the EVD outbreak, they continued providing emergency surgical care.

On July 29, 2014, EVD reached Kono. The team at KGH was initially unprepared for the outbreak and was quickly overwhelmed. Ten staff members were infected with EVD; seven died. The local population turned against the healthcare workers and blamed them for spreading the disease. Most routine health services ceased except for the isolation and care of EVD-suspected and positive patients. Initially there was limited external support and supplies, but by September, training and equipment, including personal protective equipment (PPE), began to arrive.

From September 2, 2014, until January 25, 2015, during the height of the outbreak in Kono, Drs. Marsh, Sheku, and Koedoyoma ceased all elective surgery at KGH. During that same time, however, they continued to provide emergency surgical care, which included more than 60 cesarean sections for women in obstructed labor. When asked, "Why did you do that?—No one was operating during that time." They replied, individually but with a similar humility:

- What else could we do?
- Of course we were frightened. My wife was frightened. My kids were frightened, but there was no other way out. If I left there'd be nobody on the ground and those mothers and babies would die.
- When you see a woman in obstructed labor and there's no way the baby can pass, what do you do? Leave them both to die and lose two beautiful lives? It's like asking us not to be doctors, like asking us not to breathe.

They would not stop operating, but to be as safe as possible, they worked under the assumption that everyone was EVD-positive. They protected themselves and their teams as best they could.

When elective surgery at KGH resumed, with EVD still in Sierra Leone, every surgical patient was treated as possibly EVD-positive. All fluids, blood, and tissue were treated as infectious.

It was at this time that Partners in Health (PIH), a US-based non-governmental organization, sent a team to assist at KGH. As part of the team, Andrew Michaels, a US general surgeon, deployed to assist in managing EVD cases but soon began reestablishing the surgical service.

A typical operative day, which generally also included weekends, might include several hernia repairs, some wound care, an elective cesarean section, and a smattering of other emergent cases. Emergencies consisted of incarcerated hernias, traumatic injuries, ectopic pregnancies, appendicitis, and cesarean sections for obstructed labor. The operative team consisted of a surgeon and assistant, an anesthetist, a scrub nurse, an environmental health sprayer to spray dilute chlorine solution, and additional nurses as needed. Everyone wore full PPE. From April 2014 onward, all operations at KGH were done in full category III EVD-resistant coverall suits.

The choice of specific PPE components varied, as both goggles and face shields were appropriate. Individual preferences were important because the PPE needs of a surgical team differ from those of someone working in an Ebola treatment center (ETC) or as part of a burial team. Surgical teams have added requirements for vision, manual dexterity, range of motion, and endurance of heat and stress.

The climate in the KGH operating room varied based on whether or not the air conditioning was working. The conditions were basic compared with a modern operating room in the United States or Europe, but when the electricity and air conditioning were functioning well it was more comfortable than an ETC. Unfortunately, the electricity was intermittent and the air conditioning often failed even when the power was available. It was often very hot.

We spent many hours a day in full PPE conducting operations of various complexity and duration. The only patient monitor was a pulse oximeter. Only ketamine was used for anesthesia with no intubation. There was neither electrocautery nor suction. The instrument sets were small and well used. Everything was done with a scalpel and instrument ties to save suture.

We fully donned and doffed PPE for each case. There was a significant learning curve for the safe use of PPE, especially during a surgical procedure. Avoiding dehydration was essential, as significant sweating led to the loss of fluids and electrolytes.

The healthcare workers who provided surgical care during the EVD outbreak exhibited a combination of courage and optimism. It seemed to define almost everyone, almost all of the time. The conditions were very challenging, both physically and clinically. The surgical team developed a norm of resiliency, tolerance, and humor.

The experience was both rewarding and profoundly humbling. We followed the surgeon's code. We would show up; wade through the blood and the pus together; stay until all the work was done. We learned that despite EVD being a worst-case scenario for blood-borne diseases, we could function by doing what all surgeons are trained to do, except it was a much harder, hotter, and scarier environment. The amount of trust we placed in each other as we did, case after case, was unique. It was more intimate and more compelling. We knew that if we erred, one of us would likely die.

With a shrug and a smile, from the most junior volunteer to the chief of the hospital, we managed every hardship, every frustration, every catastrophe, and every triumph with the classic mantra, "TIA: This is Africa." We said it with pride and issued it as a challenge. While the whole world hesitated, we stepped up, stood in the breach, and never looked back. "TIA." *That* is Africa.

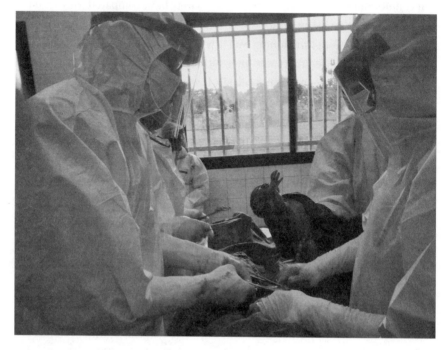

9.1. Operating during Ebola outbreak, Koidu Government Hospital, Kono, Sierra Leone. Photo courtesy Andrew J. Michaels

9

Operating in Personal Protective Equipment

ANDREW J. MICHAELS, MD, MPH, FACS, RONALD C. MARSH, MD, MIPH, MOHAMED G. SHEKU, MD, SONGOR S. J. KOEDOYOMA, MD, ANDREW M. R. HALL, DIPHE, AND KATHRYN P. BARRON, NP

In principle the use of personal protective equipment (PPE) is simple. Cover the entire body with impermeable materials, do not breach this barrier at any time, and do not allow any biological material to make contact with mucosal surfaces or skin breaks during removal. If there is any doubt about the patients or contact, assume that they are carrying Ebola virus disease (EVD) and act accordingly. That means all patients, all the time. In addition, watch out for everything and everyone. Tears in equipment, needle sticks, preventable splashes, poorly cleaned contaminated spills and equipment, and the breaches of others can all put one's life at risk.

The equipment we used to stay safe was fairly simple. Category III suits are thick plastic coveralls, essentially a hooded body suit that zips to the neck. They are waterproof for most operation room situations for about 75 minutes. Heavy rubber boots covered our feet, and we wore double gloves, a special N95 fully fitted facemask, an impermeable apron, and a full-face shield. The outer gloves were sterile, and we attended to the best aseptic techniques possible, but we did not wear sterile gowns over the PPE. All components of the PPE (except the boots) were disposed of after each use and the cost of a single full set of gear was about US$100.

One of the most critical aspects of using PPE safely is to conduct doffing (removal) correctly. Many of those who became infected with Ebola probably did so due to breaches in the doffing techniques. Proper doffing is contingent on following a prescribed procedure and not deviating from that regardless of the environmental, clinical, or mental stressors. It is inevitable that doffing will grow to be routine, and often an individual will be fatigued, even occasionally angry or frightened. Take your time and do it right every time or eventually there will be a breach. It can happen very quickly and easily. Temper your enthusiasm at being free of the suit with the realization that the water pouring down the inside of the suit is a large percentage of your precious bodily fluid and contact with the effluvia dripping down the outside of the suit could mean certain death. Take your time. It is also important to have a second person watch and make sure that the donning and doffing are done correctly.

In essence, operating in PPE is not much different from being fully gowned and gloved in a normal operating room; just much, much hotter. The recommendations for personnel working in full PPE, depending on the organization, limit the duration to between 45 minutes and 2 hours at a time and no more frequently than three times a day. There are many variables that determine the safe duration of working in PPE.

Atmospheric temperature and humidity, the age, acclimatization, and fitness of the person working, level of hydration, underlying medical issues, and the complexity of the task all affect safety in these conditions. We routinely spent between 3 and 12 hours a day in PPE, in an operating room doing relatively straightforward procedures of intermediate duration. Cases were slower because we had no electrocautery or suction and we instrument tied everything. But we did move forward through the schedule. Between cases we would doff, drink some fluids, and generally have a very rapid room turnover.

Often, if the air conditioner was working, it could be quite a reasonable experience. We would, however, begin to sweat within minutes of beginning our first case and generally continue to do so for the entire day; but this was manageable with frequent breaks and rehydration. If things got difficult we would simply play upbeat African gospel and sway. Sometimes we danced and sometimes the patient, lying on the operating room table waiting to be anesthetized, would sing and sway to the music as well.

When the generator failed it was an entirely different situation. The operating room would be lit only by indirect light coming in through large frosted windows on two sides. They were very warm and, as an afternoon progressed, the western window began to glow and radiate heat. There was no air movement inside the operating room, and within the PPE the temperature climbed rapidly in the 100% humidity environment. New factors

9.1. Lessons learned on staying safe while wearing personal protective equipment (PPE)

Don with a thought to how you will doff.

Don and doff the same way every time.

Don and doff correctly—have a safety person check your equipment and performance.

Loosen the ties on your facemask and adjust them carefully, because you cannot readjust them once you are in a hot zone.

Choose a suit that is snug enough to work in safely and loose enough to doff easily and safely.

Use the packaging bag to cover your boots when you don so they slide into the legs of your PPE more easily and do not make small tears.

Stretch the ankle elastic bands on the PPE so it comes off the boots more easily during doffing.

Some PPE suits have finger loops—do not use them. Poke a small hole in the sleeve for your thumb to prevent a gap at the cuff.

Wear long inner gloves so rundown doesn't get inside your suit if your sleeves ride up.

Try to use colored inner gloves so you can spot a tear more easily.

Tie your apron's neck up behind you so it covers up to your chin.

Goggles are more secure but fog more quickly than a face shield.

When sweat starts to pool in the sleeves of your PPE, periodically raise your arms so it runs down into your boots instead of into your gloves.

If your mask becomes so filled with sweat that you begin to suffocate, tip your head back to let it flow out—drink it if you need to. Tongue the mask off your nose and break scrub.

When you get sweat in your eyes, stay calm but step back from the table and shake it off.

Do not operate if you cannot see. You must be able to see and avoid sharps.

Do not adjust your PPE once you are in a high-risk area and NEVER allow someone else to adjust or reach inside of your PPE (to wipe sweat, for example).

Do not allow yourself to become so exhausted, dehydrated, or hot that you are at risk of fainting—doffing an unconscious colleague puts everyone at risk and is preventable.

Drink before you are thirsty and more than you can imagine. Start before you sweat and continue until your urine is clear. Do not make the ORS stronger than recommended, it will function as a bowel prep if you do and you'll lose even more fluid.

Keep a situational awareness at all times, especially for sharps and splash hazards. Rest before you become impaired and always remember—your safety depends on your actions.

Do not hesitate to break scrub if the situation feels dangerous or you are compromised.

Finally, there are no real emergencies in a hot zone—stay safe is the only absolute rule.

often entered into the operative plan. Perhaps a retractor was perfectly placed to give exposure to the field but the arm holding it blocked the light from the window. Surgeons might switch roles, not because one or the other had a better view of the far corner, but because one or the other could see at all. Sometimes we finished up by headlamp.

When operating in PPE, sweat does not simply trickle down your back but runs freely from your entire body. Your shirt dampens, clings, and then hangs heavy within minutes, and your boots begin to fill when your socks can absorb no more. The baggy space under your forearms fills with a puddle and you must raise your arms periodically so the sweat can run down into your suit and boots rather than your gloves. The inner gloves are soaked from sweaty hands anyway.

The insides of your face shield and glasses steam up, and sweat runs into your eyes, your mask, your mouth, and drips from the hanging edge of your face shield. Sometimes the mask gets so wet that you cannot breathe through it. You begin to suffocate, and when that happens you must break scrub and change your gear. It is almost impossible not to reach up and grab the mask with your hands, but you learn to use your tongue to move the mask off your nose and doff slowly. You try to step back and shake your head to clear the sweat without looking away from the field, but you are swimming by the end of a difficult case. Even when you change scrubs during the day, by evening there are many wet places that would rather be dry.

It is essential to understand that operating in PPE is not simply working in a hostile environment; it is working in a lethal environment. It is not simply the threat outside of the suit but also the conditions within that are potentially lethal. Be careful.

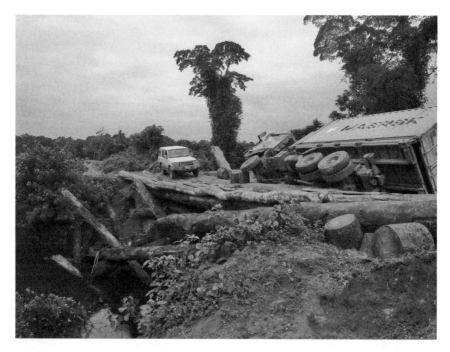

10.1. Traveling in southeastern Liberia, August, 2014. Photo courtesy Joseph Forrester

A Surgeon as Outbreak Investigator

Ebola in Liberia

JOSEPH FORRESTER, MD, MSC

I breathed in the heavy moist air. It was a smell I associated with the tropics: diesel fuel and campfire smoke, combined with the scent of flowers I did not recognize. Other times, when arriving at a new destination overseas I was filled with overwhelming excitement. But this time, and on this day, I felt different. This time I entered Liberia for the first of two deployments as an Epidemic Intelligence Service (EIS) officer of the US Centers for Disease Control and Prevention (CDC) just as Ebola virus disease (EVD) was spreading throughout the country. It was July 23, 2014.

At this time, EVD was already confirmed in Monrovia, the capital, and in Lofa County, in the north along the Guinea border. Information from other areas was limited, often just rumors or presumptions. There were no reliable reports about what was actually happening on the ground in the other counties. Cases were reported in Bong and Nimba Counties, northeast of Monrovia, but specifics were vague. Of concern was the increasing proportion of suspected cases that were laboratory-confirmed. This suggested that many more positive cases were undocumented.

The first night, I was assigned to travel to Bong and Nimba Counties to obtain detailed information about the extent of the outbreak. We left early in the morning and after a few hours arrived at Phebe Hospital in Gbarnga.

Phebe Hospital is a regional referral center for Bong County. The facility has approximately 200 inpatient beds occupied by 100 to 125 patients at any given time. What we found was disturbing. The hospital was empty. The day before we arrived, all the staff and patients had left the hospital over fear of EVD.

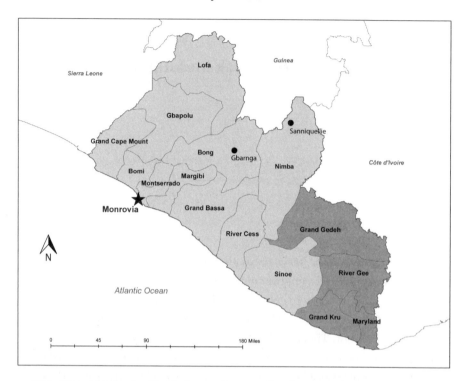

10.2. Map of Liberia. Shaded counties are the four southeastern counties assessed. County capital Monrovia marked with star. Bong County capital Gbarnga and Nimba County capital Sanniquellie marked with dots. Courtesy of CDC

In the prior week, five nurses and nurses' aides were infected and died of EVD. One physician was also infected, and luckily he survived. The index case who spread EVD to the Phebe Hospital staff was a young woman who had traveled from Lofa County after exposure to EVD there. At that time, the stigma surrounding EVD was rampant and misinformation was circulating faster than the disease. The index patient had not told the staff her true name and neither divulged her high-risk exposure nor her travel history. As a result, the staff did not use strict infection precautions and were exposed.

Our footsteps echoed through the deserted hallways as we toured the hospital with the medical director. It was as if everyone working and receiving care had just vanished. Work was left on desks, flowers left in flowerpots, and charts left on the racks. But the most important parts of the hospital, the patients and the staff, had vanished.

The abandonment of Phebe Hospital was concerning, but even more disturbing were the healthcare consequences. Patients now had no access to modern therapies. Traditional healers without proper training, medicine, painkillers, or antibiotics would treat any surgical or medical emergency. Luckily for pregnant women C.B. Dunbar Maternity Hospital was still functioning and providing emergency obstetric services. But the medical director was concerned. Patient admissions had decreased. There was fear among patients that healthcare workers were transmitting the virus and fear among healthcare workers that the facilities were contaminated. In August, both Phebe and C. B. Dunbar Hospitals would close, leaving residents of the area without any option for formal healthcare.

I am a surgery resident. I am in training. I have a compulsion to want to fix problems. When I encounter a patient with appendicitis, I want to cut the appendix out. When I see a health facility functionally disintegrate, I want to step in and help. But since I am an EIS officer, that was not my role. It was a role-reversal that I struggled with throughout my deployment. On my visit to Bong and Nimba Counties I was sent to gather information about the outbreak, to help provide support to the public health team, and to report back so that national-level public health decisions could be made. So, less than 48 hours after arriving in Bong County, I headed to Nimba County. I was concerned with what we would find.

We visited G. W. Harvey Hospital located at the county seat in Sanniquellie. The hospital had just over 50 beds and was the referral center for Nimba County. In the weeks prior to our arrival the staff had cared for at least four EVD patients. But without personal protective equipment (PPE) and training, the healthcare workers had stopped working. Similar to Phebe Hospital, all staff and patients had initially left, though when we visited some had recently returned. We were told there was currently a patient with suspected EVD in isolation.

Still somewhat naive about the lack of preparation in the country, we walked with the public health officer down the hallway and stood outside the isolation room. Just then, the door opened, and the potentially infected patient stumbled out, several feet from us. I stood in amazement and fear. The nurse at the end of the hall, sitting in partial PPE, stood up, and walked past us. She was wearing street shoes, a Tyvek jumpsuit, gloves, and a surgical mask but no eye protection. She caught the patient and returned her to her room. Without changing PPE or washing her hands, the same nurse then walked right next door into the mother-baby room to administer care. I watched aghast, frozen in place, unable to respond.

This was but one example of the magnitude of the challenges faced by the Liberian healthcare system at the start of the outbreak. Healthcare workers were present but generally not adequately trained. PPE was available in limited quantities at some facilities but not enough to be effective. Some hospitals were able to remain functional but without the training or PPE that would allow them to function safely. In many instances, the lack of training and inconsistent PPE usage contributed to a false sense of security among healthcare workers, which possibly resulted in exposure to EVD.

Returning to Monrovia we attempted to process the events of the previous several days. Liberia, which was emerging from decades of political instability and violence, was faced with an EVD outbreak, and the country's healthcare infrastructure was ill prepared to deal with such an overwhelming threat. On that rainy car ride through the muddy roads, my mind was overwhelmed with thoughts: Had the virus mutated? Was it more contagious than was thought? Could I have been, or would I be, exposed without knowing it?

Back in the city, by the area known as Cement Factory Town, we saw a body lying bloated in a puddle of water. At this point, the number of dead and dying victims exceeded the capacity for safe burials. As a surgery resident and physician, I have witnessed people die. Seeing death is never easy for me, but somehow, when people die in a trauma bay or in a hospital, I have a sense of control despite the chaos. Seeing people die in the streets, left alone in the sun, dehumanized, was entirely different. There is no level of training adequate for such sights. Over the coming months, seeing these bodies became commonplace.

My second assignment was to investigate how two US healthcare workers had become infected at the Eternal Love Winning Africa (ELWA) Hospital run by the US nongovernmental organization (NGO) Samaritan's Purse. I visited the hospital. It was at that time abandoned. I took notes as I toured the facility. An Ebola treatment unit (ETU) had been created out of a chapel, and a cross still remained on the outside of the building. A white tarpaulin weathered by the elements lay flaccid in the light rain.

That night I got back to my hotel room exhausted. "Ebola paranoia," a fear that I had been exposed to Ebola, took hold. It was an irrational fear, but it was strong. In the shower, I poured a bleach solution over my body. Invisible, deadly adversaries wreaked havoc with my mind. That night EVD had won.

Nevertheless, over the following days we organized the notes from interviews and site visits about the exposures at ELWA Hospital. Slowly, it became apparent that the strict culture of safety in the ETU did not extend to the less recognized, but equally high-risk settings of the hospital emergency department and triage area. Findings from this investigation would later provide guidance to healthcare providers and help ETUs remain staffed, functional, and safe.

Around this time, rumors circulated of EVD cases in southeastern Liberia. Based on my visit to Bong and Nimba Counties, I was concerned that the southeast would also be ill prepared. We needed to know how far the outbreak had spread and what could be done to stop it. I went to investigate not knowing what to expect.

Traveling overland underscored the challenges Liberia faced in responding to the outbreak. A distance that would take half-a-day to drive in the United States required many days of hard driving. By early August, the rainy season was in full force and dirt roads were muddy and often impassible. Bridges constructed by the logging companies broke down quickly in the tropical environment. During the hours and days I spent in our Land Cruiser, I could not help but wonder what impact effective and safe transportation would have had on our ability to respond to the outbreak. If we could get patients transported more rapidly, we could get them into an ETU faster, improve their outcome, and protect healthcare workers. If we could just get samples to the labs quickly, we could identify patients and perform more effective triage. But the same barriers to transportation that were hampering our ability to respond quickly to the outbreak were also the barriers that prevented EVD from spreading even faster.

Unfortunately, the status of healthcare in the four southeastern Liberian counties of Grand Gedeh, Grand Kru, River Gee, and Maryland was similar to what I found in Bong and Nimba. I evaluated three of four referral hospitals for the area, which essentially provided all inpatient and operative services for a population of 386,000 people. In two of the four hospitals, there were no nurses, as they had stopped coming to work. Prior to EVD, there were six physicians for these two counties, but by the time I surveyed the facilities, only three remained; the others either left or died.

In all the facilities, nursing students, nursing aids, and community health volunteers were helping provide basic and emergency medical services, including emergency surgery and obstetric care. Medical supplies were limited. Stocks of nonsterile and sterile gloves were depleted or absent at each facility. Hand washing stations were rarely available in the hospitals, let alone at checkpoints throughout the counties. In many areas, hollowed out bamboo was used to hold water, which could then be used for hand washing.

Stigma was also spreading quickly in southeastern Liberia. Healthcare workers were reporting increasing animosity outside of their work environment over concerns that they were spreading the disease. The healthcare workers I met with were in a no-win situation; they were stigmatized through their work, they did not have adequate protection, and they did not receive adequate training.

Throughout the deployment, I reflected on the parallels between Camus's novel, The Plague, and the EVD outbreak. The healthcare workers dealt with fear, death, and uncertainty daily. But as Camus wrote, "They knew now that if there is one thing one can always yearn for, and sometimes attain, it is human love." Despite the risks, and the fear, and the uncertainty, many of the remaining healthcare workers were still caring, still showing compassion. It was as true a demonstration of selfless care for another suffering human as I have witnessed.

But despite the best intentions of these healthcare workers, the investigation provided a bleak assessment of the capacity for these counties to deal with persons infected with EVD. The infrastructure to distribute PPE, to ensure its appropriate use through widespread training of health workers, and to maintain basic medical services was not there. I ended this first deployment with much uncertainty about the outbreak response.

In November 2014, I had the opportunity to redeploy to Liberia for a second CDC mission. At this point the exponential transmission of EVD had slowed. Also, more ETUs were established, stigma and misinformation surrounding EVD was decreasing, and the outbreak was slowly coming under control. Among other tasks during this second deployment, I was encouraged to work with the Liberian Ministry of Health and Social Welfare (LMoHSW) to restore basic healthcare services in Monrovia.

Approximately 1 million people live in Monrovia, and even at the worst of the epidemic more people were dying every day from commonly encountered medical conditions than were dying from EVD. In July and August, health facilities had closed; there was no capacity to effectively triage, identify, isolate, and treat patients with EVD. This contributed to the devastating impact that the outbreak had on the healthcare system. But as the capacity to isolate and treat patients with EVD improved during October and November, an equally chilling problem became apparent: how to safely and effectively restore basic healthcare services.

Thankfully, at this time, I was able to work with personnel from the LMoHSW, various NGOs, and the World Health Organization (WHO). Broadly our goal was to reduce and eventually eliminate the opportunity for EVD infection among healthcare workers. Only by ensuring that healthcare workers could practice in a safe environment would trust, both among healthcare workers and the general public, be restored. My role in attaining this goal was twofold: (1) ensure that a basic infection prevention package (triage, PPE, and training) was available at every facility in Monrovia; and (2) develop a protocol to rapidly audit health facilities that had an infected healthcare worker.

To ensure that every health facility had infection prevention coverage, we first needed to make sure that we were aware of all the facilities in Monrovia. While LMoHSW knew about the public facilities, many private facilities were unknown. Working with LMoHSW, we partner-mapped all 290 healthcare facilities in Monrovia for an accurate and up-to-date list. We then convened a meeting of the NGOs participating in infection prevention activities in the city. Over several hours we spoke about each facility to determine which NGOs were active where. This ensured that every facility had at least one NGO capable of confirming a functioning triage system, availability of PPE, and appropriately trained staff. While this was a seemingly small intervention, it enabled us (LMoHSW, NGOs, CDC, and WHO) to operate in concert, minimizing duplication of efforts and making provision of support as efficient as possible in an otherwise chaotic environment.

My second task was to work with the LMoHSW and WHO to develop a protocol to evaluate a health facility that had an infected healthcare worker. On November 8, 2014, the US military finished construction of the Monrovia Medical Unit (MMU), a center designed to care for EVD-infected healthcare workers. A by-product of this centralized care for healthcare workers was that the LMoHSW could more efficiently track which healthcare workers became infected, and as important, what facilities they came from. After identifying the facility with an infected healthcare worker, a structured audit was administered with the goal of identifying potential exposure sources.

Identifying problem areas at a facility is important, but determining ways to address and fix them is even more so. We had to leverage NGO support to impart lasting educational and structural change at these facilities; we needed to reduce the chance that another healthcare worker would get exposed in the future. By the time my second deployment was ending in late December, we had successfully put our protocol to use and were able to audit two such facilities. The simple interventions we organized (basic shelter for triage, sustainable barrier precaution equipment, and training) allowed healthcare workers at these facilities to resume patient care activities, and do so in a way that they, and their future patients, felt protected.

I was privileged, with my two deployments, to spend over three months in Liberia assisting in the EVD response. I saw an outbreak take hold of a country, but I also saw the remarkable resolve of people to fight through incredible adversity to provide care for fellow humans. Epidemics have been, and will continue to be, one of the greatest challenges faced by humanity. Gone are the days where an outbreak in one area of the world would burn in isolation. Rapid international travel, intertwined global economies, and near-instantaneous reporting ensure that outbreaks have rapid and powerful social, economic, and medical impacts. EVD highlighted flaws in our ability to respond to international epidemic threats. We would be wise to learn from this experience and work to develop an international response force capable of identifying, controlling, and resolving the inevitable epidemics of the future.

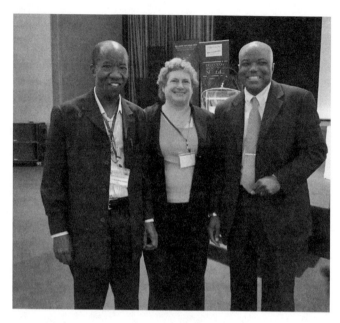

C.1. Thaim B. Kamara, MBBS, FWACS, from Sierra Leone (*left*), Sherry M. Wren, MD, FACS, FCS(ECSA), from the United States (*center*), and Lawrence Sherman, MD, FWACS, from Liberia (*right*) after presenting on Ebola at the West African College of Surgeons annual meeting held in Abidjan, Côte d'Ivoire. March 2015. Photo courtesy Sherry M. Wren

Conclusion

SHERRY M. WREN, MD, FACS, FCS(ECSA),
AND ADAM L. KUSHNER, MD, MPH, FACS

Although the World Health Organization officially declared the West African Ebola virus disease (EVD) outbreak over on January 14, 2016, a few hours later, EVD-positive patients were reported in Sierra Leone. Given the difficulties in transportation, communication, and the weak health surveillance system, pockets of cases or even full outbreaks are likely to recur.

Will EVD truly ever be eradicated? That is difficult to say. There are now rapid EVD tests and promising EVD vaccine trials underway. Hopefully in the coming months and years the threat of EVD will recede. Yet, we must not forget the lessons that this outbreak taught us, lessons that are important for dealing with EVD and perhaps other infectious diseases. With increasing globalization and better local transportation and infrastructure, outbreaks that in the past were contained in relative isolation now easily spread to cities and beyond.

EVD may return to West Africa or elsewhere, other infectious diseases, such as Middle East respiratory syndrome (MERS) or Zika may affect thousands. Not all of these diseases will have surgical components, but surgeons should be at the table when planning and interventions are discussed. At the 68th World Health Assembly in 2015, surgical care was finally officially recognized as an important part of healthcare. Surgeons must step forward, and the public health community must recognize the needs of surgical patients, something that continues to be woefully lacking in international discussions about emerging infectious disease outbreaks.

As of November 2016 there are still no official guidelines discussing approaches to surgical patients during an EVD outbreak. Meanwhile specific guidelines exist for breast-feeding, hemodialysis, pregnancy, aerosol-generating procedures, and safe injection practices. Basic surgical care needs must also be addressed.

From the perspective of surgical care and operative experiences, remembering lessons learned and educating future providers about EVD is vital. During the West African outbreak the establishment of guidelines and protocols to safeguard healthcare workers was an important initial part of the fight. Proper techniques for safely donning and doffing personal protective equipment (PPE) had to be taught and learned. In addition, just as panic and stigma needed to be addressed during the initial days of AIDS, so too were safe and logical methods needed to care for EVD patients and protect those who cared for them.

In this book, frontline healthcare workers in the United States and in West Africa describe their experiences with EVD from a surgical and procedure-based perspective. The three sections look at a view from the United States, a view from Sierra Leone, and technical considerations and beyond.

As surgeons who worked alongside local colleagues in West Africa, we have seen firsthand the inadequacies of the healthcare system. District hospitals often have no running water or power, simple procedures such as inserting chest tubes cannot be performed due to a lack of skilled personnel or simple equipment or sterile supplies. Eye protection and gloves are often in short supply. The rapid spread of EVD was in some way not surprising. Sadly, the many resources needed to care for EVD-infected or suspected patients, even though they are similar to the prevention of the spread of HIV or other blood-borne diseases, were mostly unavailable.

What the EVD outbreak also showed us was that death and disability do not just occur from the infectious complications of the virus. As healthcare worker after healthcare worker succumbed to EVD, the local population lost trust in the health providers and the health facilities. Hundreds or thousands of other preventable deaths and disabilities most likely occurred from simple wounds and injuries, obstructed labor, or conditions such as incarcerated hernias or appendicitis that went untreated. We will never know the full extent of these non-EVD deaths.

As we look toward the future, it is important to recognize that providing surgical care is more than having a surgeon. Surgical care consists of safe anesthesia, nurses, and cleaners. The teams that were involved in burials or the community health workers who visited each and every community were important as well. Surgical care also necessitates sterile supplies and equipment, as well as patient education to ensure timely presentations while care can be rendered.

Watching the outbreak develop from afar, but also seeing the effect on our own hospitals and communities in the United States, brought us to see the necessity for this book. We needed to document why we sought to develop Surgery and Ebola guidelines (Chapter 1). The teamwork and preparation of the Nebraska Biocontainment Unit provided great insights into what was possible with political will and sufficient resources, but it also showed that the system is not perfect. Without timely referral, not everyone can be saved (Chapter 2).

We sought to document personal reflections and the health system collapse (Chapters 3, 4, 5, and 6). These chapters describe the pain of having to close a maternity hospital in light of the risks and benefits to staff and patients, the death of clinical officer trainees, and a massive decrease in surgical caseloads.

We also wanted to document the successes. How teams from Partners In Health and Kings College worked alongside Sierra Leonean healthcare workers to improve systems, develop protocols, and subsequently save lives and make things better (Chapters 7, 8, 9, and 10).

Despite an initial grim prognosis (Chapters 3, 4, and 5), pregnant women with EVD survived, as did their children (Chapter 7). What initially seemed unimaginable became routine.

This book is a collection of personal stories and insights from the growing group of healthcare professionals with experience treating EVD-positive patients. Though we hope another EVD outbreak will not occur, we must consider the possibility and prepare for the future. We must work as a team, remember the lessons learned, and prepare for the future. The goal must be to move from despair to hope.

ADDITIONAL READING

Gupta S, Wong EG, Kushner AL. Scarcity of protective items against HIV and other bloodborne infections in 13 low- and middle-income countries. *Trop Med Int Health.* 2014 Nov;19(11):1384-90.

Index